Learning About Agitation, Confusion, and Altered Mental Status

A Programmed Text

Theodore A. Stern, MD

Learning About Agitation, Confusion, and Altered Mental Status

A Programmed Text

Learning About Agitation, Confusion, and Altered Mental Status: A Programmed Text

ISBN-13: 978-0-9991483-8-9 (print)
ISBN-13: 978-0-9991483-7-2 (ebook)

Book Production: Dianne Russell, Octal Productions, LLC
Copyeditor: Bob Russell, Octal Publishing, LLC
Cover Design: Falcone Creative Design, LLC
Book Design: Dianne Russell, Octal Productions, LLC
Printing and Binding: RP Graphics
Production Managers: Jane Pimental and Grace Shanks, MGH Psychiatry Academy
This book is printed on acid-free paper.

To lifelong learners across multiple disciplines.

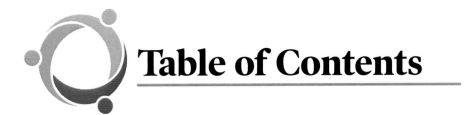

Table of Contents

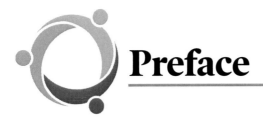

Preface

Have you ever wondered why people become confused? Have you ever been perplexed by how best to treat agitation? Have you ever thought that it might be better to prevent delirium than to treat it?

Altered mental status (involving agitation, confusion, and perceptual disturbances) is a topic of concern for clinicians of all specialties. Learning **who** is at risk for an altered mental status, **what** we can say or do to prevent or to treat individuals with an altered mental status, **why** people become agitated or confused, and **how** we can assess and treat alterations of mental status is key to providing timely treatment and saving lives.

To assess your knowledge about this subject, a pre-test is provided.

After taking this pre-test, move directly to the text (**without checking the answer key** at the end of the book).

Next, read the programmed text. It provides you with an opportunity for layered learning, with information offered in bite-sized bits. After each section, fill in the missing words (indicated by blanks) with the correct answer; this enables you to build knowledge in small steps. You will learn better if you do not look at the answers before you fill in the missing words. Therefore, cover up the answer adjacent to each section using the supplied *bookmark* (found at the back of this book), until you have filled in the missing words.

This format makes this volume appear incredibly simple; nevertheless, completing this step-by-step workbook will help you achieve working knowledge about the assessment and management of altered mental status.

Follow the instructions; skipping sections will interfere with the learning process. You can complete the tests and read the text in one sitting.

After completing the entire text, take the post-reading test. This helps you assess how much you have learned from this exercise.

Then, score your pre-test and post-reading test to determine your raw score and percentage of correct responses so that you can see how much you learned.

Enjoy the painless process.

Theodore A. Stern, MD

Pre-Reading Quiz

Pre-Reading Quiz: Answer Sheet

1. _____

2. _____

3. _____

4. _____

5. _____

6. _____

7. _____

8. _____

9. _____

10. _____

11. _____

12. _____

13. _____

14. _____

15. _____

16. _____

17. _____

18. _____

19. _____

20. _____

21. _____

22. _____

23. _____

24. _____

25. _____

26. _____

27. _____

28. _____

29. _____

30. _____

31. _____

32. _____

33. _____

34. _____

35. _____

36. _____

37. _____

38. _____

39. _____

40. _____

41. _____

42. _____

43. _____

44. _____

45. _____

46. _____

47. _____

48. _____

49. _____

50. _____

Pre-Reading Quiz: Questions

1. Which of the following is the best term to describe a clinician's bedside assessment of affect, behavior, and cognition?
   A. Disability assessment
   B. Mental status examination
   C. Neuropsychiatric testing
   D. Physical examination

2. Which of the following is assessed when a clinician observes how a patient appears?
   A. Affect
   B. Cognition
   C. Judgment
   D. Mood

3. Which of the following is assessed when a clinician asks a patient how they are feeling?
   A. Affect
   B. Cognition
   C. Judgment
   D. Mood

4. Acute brain failure is most closely related to which of the following terms?
   A. Binswanger's encephalopathy
   B. Delirium
   C. Dementia
   D. Seizures

5. Chronic brain failure is most closely related to which of the following terms?
   A. Delirium
   B. Dementia
   C. Hypoglycemia
   D. Seizures

6. Which of the following features is characteristic of delirium?
   A. Abulia
   B. Agnosia
   C. Aphasia
   D. Disorientation

7. Which of the following features is characteristic of delirium?
   A. Impaired attention and concentration
   B. Non-fluent aphasia
   C. Nystagmus
   D. Word-finding difficulty

8. Which of the following features is characteristic of delirium?
   A. Negativism
   B. Perceptual disturbances
   C. Staring spells
   D. Waxy flexibility

9. Paranoid ideas are an example of which of the following?
   A. Thought blocking
   B. Thought broadcasting
   C. Thought content
   D. Thought process

10. Which of the following terms best describes excessive, non-purposeful motor activity?

   A. Agitation

   B. Catatonia

   C. Delirium

   D. Psychosis

11. Which of the following terms is used to describe the task of asking a patient to subtract the number seven sequentially from 100?

   A. Concrete thinking

   B. Executive function

   C. Planning

   D. Serial sevens

12. Which of the following is the domain tested by asking a patient to spell the word "WORLD" backward?

   A. Abulia

   B. Attention and concentration

   C. Broca's aphasia

   D. Wernicke's aphasia

13. Which of the following is a brief test of cognition?

   A. HAM-D

   B. MMPI

   C. MMSE

   D. PHQ-9

14. Which of the following is a brief test of cognition?
    A. MoCA
    B. PAI
    C. WAIS
    D. WCST

15. Which of the following is a brief test of cognition?
    A. BPRS
    B. CAM-ICU
    C. CGI
    D. MINI

16. On average, how many minutes does it take to administer the MMSE?
    A. Less than two
    B. 5 to 10
    C. 15 to 20
    D. 45 to 60

17. Which of the following is a normal score on the MoCA?
    A. Less than 10
    B. 10 to 15
    C. 20 to 25
    D. More than 26

18. Which of the following can be assessed by poor placement of numbers when a patient is asked to draw a clock?
    A. Aprosodia
    B. Broca's aphasia
    C. Executive dysfunction
    D. Wernicke's syndrome

19. Which of the following terms describes seeing something that isn't there?
    A. A delusion
    B. A hallucination
    C. An illusion
    D. A paranoid belief

20. Which of the following terms would best describe the experience of a patient with a Foley catheter, when he tells you that he sees a snake sitting on his leg?
    A. A delusion
    B. A hallucination
    C. An illusion
    D. A paranoid belief

21. Which of the following is the most important determinant of the treatment of the agitated and delirious patient?
    A. Age of the patient
    B. Cost of the treatment
    C. Etiology of the delirium
    D. Prognosis of the patient

22. Which of the following is the *least* helpful term in establishing an etiology of delirium?
    A. Hypoglycemia
    B. Hypponatremia
    C. Hypoxemia
    D. ICU psychosis

23. Which of the following terms is most synonymous with word "delirious"?
    A. Agitated
    B. Encephalopathic
    C. Paranoid
    D. Psychotic

24. Which of the following is a characteristic feature of delirium?
    A. Fever
    B. Fluctuations
    C. Paranoia
    D. Persistence

25. Which of the following best describes a fixed, false belief?
    A. A delusion
    B. An illusion
    C. A hallucination
    D. Paranoia

26. Which of the following is most closely associated with the development of mania?
    A. Beta blockers
    B. Calcium channel-blockers
    C. Corticosteroids
    D. NSAIDs

27. Which of the following mnemonics can be used to recall the life-threatening causes of delirium?
    A. DIGFAST
    B. DTRHIGH
    C. SIGECAPS
    D. WWHHHHIIMMPS

28. The triad of ataxia, confusion, and ophthalmoplegia is highly suggestive of which of the following conditions?
    A. Catatonia
    B. Delirium
    C. Serotonin syndrome
    D. Wernicke's encephalopathy

29. Which of the following would be most likely if a patient demonstrates confusion, tachycardia, mydriasis, reduced bowel sounds, dry skin, and flushing?
    A. Adrenergic excess
    B. Anticholinergic delirium
    C. Hypoglycemia
    D. Narcotic withdrawal

30. Which of the following can reverse many of the manifestations of an amitriptyline overdose?
    A. Atropine
    B. Flumazenil
    C. Naloxone
    D. Physostigmine

31. Deficiency of which of the following substances would be likely to lead to Wernicke's encephalopathy?
    A. Folic acid
    B. Niacin
    C. Thiamine
    D. Vitamin B_{12}

32. Benzodiazepines with which of the following half-lives are most likely to lead to a withdrawal syndrome after sudden discontinuation or a dramatic decrease in the dose?

    A. Less than three hours

    B. 5 to 10 hours

    C. 10 to 20 hours

    D. More than 40 hours

33. Which of the following routes of administration of haloperidol is likely to lead to the lowest risk of acute extrapyramidal symptoms?

    A. Intramuscular

    B. Intravenous

    C. Oral

    D. Transdermal patch

34. Dementia is a syndrome characterized by a clinically significant decline in memory as well as by at least one of the following domains?

    A. Ambulation

    B. Appetite

    C. Higher cortical function

    D. Mood

35. Dementia usually develops over which of the following time periods?

    A. Minutes to hours

    B. Days to weeks

    C. Weeks to months

    D. Months to years

36. Dementia is manifest by which of the following?
    A. A tripling of the prevalence every five years beyond the age of 60
    B. An acquired decline in memory
    C. An irreversible loss of memory
    D. Weight gain

37. The prevalence of dementia in individuals above the age of 60 is which of the following?
    A. 1%
    B. 5%
    C. 15%
    D. 50%

38. The prevalence of dementia at age 60 is which of the following?
    A. 1%
    B. 5%
    C. 15%
    D. 50%

39. The prevalence of dementia among those aged 85 is which of the following?
    A. 5%
    B. 15%
    C. 50%
    D. 75%

40. In which of the following conditions is there an autosomal dominant pattern of inheritance of dementia?
    A. Diffuse Lewy body disease
    B. Huntington's disease
    C. Multiple sclerosis
    D. Parkinson's disease

41. Which of the following types of dementia is associated with a step-wise decline in function?
    A. Alzheimer's disease
    B. Diffuse Lewy body disease
    C. Parkinson's disease
    D. Vascular dementia

42. Which of the following is identified as an activity of daily living?
    A. Toileting
    B. Managing money
    C. Shopping
    D. Using the telephone

43. Which of the following is identified as an instrumental activity of daily living?
    A. Bathing
    B. Dressing
    C. Feeding
    D. Preparing meals

44. Which of the following statements about Alzheimer's disease is *true*?
    A. Afflicted patients are not allowed to sign contracts
    B. Remote memory is worse than recent memory
    C. Symptom onset is abrupt
    D. The course is gradually progressive

45. The presence of headache and malaise in someone with cognitive impairment should suggest which of the following conditions?

A. A degenerative disease

B. Obstructive hydrocephalus

C. Pseudodementia

D. Vasculitis

46. The presence of ataxia, incontinence, and confusion should suggest which of the following conditions?

A. AIDS

B. Normal pressure hydrocephalus

C. Parkinson's disease

D. Syphilis

47. The presence of extrapyramidal symptoms should suggest which of the following conditions?

A. Alzheimer's disease

B. Diffuse Lewy body disease

C. Normal pressure hydrocephalus

D. Vitamin B_{12} deficiency

48. Which of the following is an autoimmune disorder associated with cognitive impairment?

A. Creutzfeldt-Jacob disease

B. Lyme disease

C. Neurosyphilis

D. Systemic lupus erythematosus

49. Which of the following is a brief bedside cognitive screening test?

  A. "Draw-a-clock" test
  B. HAM-D
  C. SCID
  D. YBOCS

50. Which of the following is the phrase associated with the concept that a patient can have multiple simultaneous conditions?

  A. Bernoulli's theorem
  B. Hickam's dictum
  C. Markovnikov's rule
  D. Occam's razor

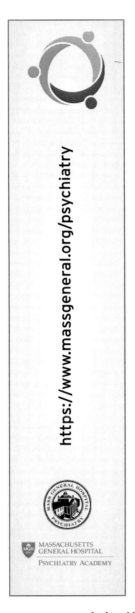

Cover the answers as you take the pre-test by using the bookmark (shown here) found at the back of this book.

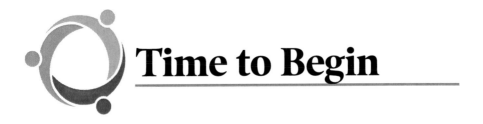# Time to Begin

Remember to fill in the missing words (indicated by the blank spaces) before you look at the answers (i.e., in the shaded area adjacent to the text).

Enjoy the process.

Acute changes in affect (i.e., how someone appears), behavior (i.e., how someone acts), and cognition (i.e., how someone thinks) can be assessed by performing a mental status assessment or mental status examination.

An examination of how someone looks, acts, and thinks is called the _____ _____ _____.

mental; status examination

Changes in affect, behavior, and cognition may indicate an acute alteration in medical and neurological functions (e.g., low blood pressure, anemia, low blood sugar, infection) or reflect a chronic condition (e.g., dementia).

Changes in behavior and cognition can result from new-onset changes in medical or neurological conditions (e.g., delirium) or from those that are _____, as in dementia.

chronic

Assessment of mental status via the mental status examination can lead to diagnosis of a life-threatening condition; for example, delirium. Making a diagnosis of delirium can facilitate timely treatment. Timely treatment typically prevents further complications and longer hospital stays.

Timely _____ can prevent further complications associated with conditions that cause delirium.

treatment

Alterations in mental status that are found in delirium often include impaired attention and memory, restlessness, agitation, disorganized thinking, disorientation (e.g., not knowing the date, the time, the place), as well as illusions (i.e., misperceptions of something that one sees, hears, or feels), hallucinations (e.g., perceptions of what you hear, see, feel, taste, or smell but that aren't really there), delusions (i.e., firm and unshakeable beliefs that something is true when it is untrue), and disrupted sleep patterns (e.g., being awake at night and asleep during the day or sleeping too much or too little).

Alterations in mental status that are found in delirium often include impaired attention and memory, restlessness, agitation, disorganized thinking, _____ (e.g., not knowing the date, the time, the place), as well as _____ (i.e., misperceptions of something that one sees, hears, or feels), hallucinations (e.g., perceptions of what you hear, see, feel, taste, or smell but that aren't really there), delusions (i.e., firm and unshakeable beliefs that something is true when it is untrue), and disrupted sleep patterns (e.g., being awake at night and asleep during the day or sleeping too much or too little).

disorientation

illusions

The hallmarks of delirium are impaired attention and concentration, disorientation, and perceptual disturbances (e.g., illusions or hallucinations).

The hallmarks of delirium are impaired _____ and _____, disorientation, and perceptual disturbances (e.g., illusions or hallucinations).

attention
concentration

Acute changes in affect, behavior, and cognition (aka the ABCs) among hospitalized patients require timely recognition and effective treatment.

Acute changes in affect, behavior, and _____ among hospitalized patients require timely recognition (regarding its presence and its cause) and effective treatment.

cognition

Assessment of appearance, behavior, attention, language, vocabulary, orientation, memory, thought processes (e.g., whether thoughts are connected logically), thought content (e.g., paranoid ideas) and judgment comprise the mental status examination.

Assessment of appearance, behavior, attention, language, vocabulary, orientation, memory, thought _____ (e.g., whether thoughts are connected logically), thought _____ (e.g., paranoid ideas) and judgment comprise the mental status examination.

processes
content

The mental status examination can be completed in several minutes, even if the patient is critically ill and is receiving intensive care.

The mental status examination can be completed in several _____, even if the patient is critically ill and is receiving intensive care.

minutes

Delirium is a dread complication of many medical and surgical conditions and their treatments.

An acute complication of medical and surgical conditions and their treatments that can be called acute brain failure is _____.

delirium

Delirium can be manifest by disturbances of attention, orientation, memory, and sleep, as well as by agitation and hallucinations.

Delirium can be manifest by disturbances of _____, _____, _____, and sleep, as well as by agitation and hallucinations.

attention; orientation; memory

Agitation (manifest by excessive, usually non-purposeful motor activity, and internal tension) can vary in intensity from a state of mild restlessness to one of violent combativeness.

High degrees of _____ can jeopardize a patient's health and threaten the stability of a patient's cardiovascular status.

agitation

If left untreated, agitation or delirium can also jeopardize the safety of patients and staff.

If left untreated, agitation or delirium can also jeopardize the safety of patients and _____.

staff

At the very least, agitation can be a nuisance to staff, which can sap their emotional and physical resources.

At the very least, agitation can be a nuisance to staff, which can sap their _____ and _____ resources.

emotional; physical

Affect, appearance (how is the patient appears to you), and behavior are important features of the mental status examination.

Affect, _____ (how is the patient appears to you), and behavior are important features of the mental status examination.

appearance

Descriptors of agitated individuals often includes terms such as agitated, fidgety, restless, uncooperative, and irritable.

Terms such as agitated, fidgety, _____, uncooperative, and irritable are often used to describe an agitated patient.

restless

Attention and concentration ability are typically impaired by delirium.

Attention and concentration ability are typically _____ by delirium.

impaired

Attention and concentration ability can be assessed by asking the patient to spell the word "WORLD" backward, or to subtract the number seven from 100 and from the number generated by the subtraction (e.g., 100, 93, 86, 79, 72, 65...), a task labeled as "serial sevens."

Subtracting the number seven from 100 and from the number generated by the subtraction (e.g., 100, 93, 86, 79, 72, 65...) is a task labeled as "performing _____."

serial sevens

Attention and concentration ability can also be assessed by asking the patient to spell the word "_____" backward, which involves concentrating on the recall of five letters in a set order.

WORLD

Several screening tests and tools are available for the assessment of cognition; these tests include the Mini-Mental State Examination (MMSE). the Montreal Cognitive Assessment (MoCA), and the Confusion Assessment Method for the ICU (CAM-ICU).

Screening tests for the assessment of cognition include the Mini-Mental State Examination (MMSE), the _____ _____ _____ (MoCA), and the Confusion Assessment Method for the ICU (CAM-ICU).

Montreal; Cognitive; Assessment

Each of these tests is easy to administer and to score. Each assesses a variety of cognitive domains (e.g., attention, memory, language, planning, orientation) that reflect function of different brain territories.

Each of these tests is easy to _____ and to _____. Each assesses a variety of cognitive domains (e.g., to assess orientation to time and place, registration, attention, calculation, recall, language, repetition, the ability to follow complex commands) that reflect function of different brain territories.

administer
score

The MMSE asks questions that help to evaluate orientation to time and place, registration, attention, calculation, recall, language, repetition, and the ability to follow complex commands. Five points can be given for orientation to time and for orientation to place.

Five points can be given for orientation to time and for _____ to place.

orientation

The MMSE, created by Folstein and colleagues in 1975, has a maximum score of 30 points. It can be used to provide a crude assessment of cognition and a tool to track the course of cognition over time.

It takes roughly 5 to 10 minutes to administer.

The MMSE takes roughly _____ to _____ minutes to administer.

5
10

Unfortunately, the MMSE is not particularly sensitive in its ability to detect mild cognitive impairment and it does not reliably distinguish those with Alzheimer's disease from people without dementia.

Unfortunately, the MMSE is not particularly sensitive in its ability to detect _____ _____ _____ and it does not reliably distinguish those with Alzheimer's disease from people _____ _____.

mild; cognitive
impairment
without
dementia

The MoCA test is another 30-point test that can be administered in less than 10 minutes.

The MoCA test is another 30-point test that can be administered in less than _____ minutes.   10

The MoCA assesses several different cognitive domains, including short-term memory, visual spatial function, executive function (e.g., planning, sequencing), attention, concentration ability, working memory, language, and orientation to time and place.

The MoCA assesses several different cognitive domains, including short-term _____, visual spatial function, executive function (e.g., planning, sequencing), attention, _____ ability, working memory, language, and _____ to time and place.

memory

concentration
orientation

Scores on the MoCA of 26 and higher are generally considered as normal.

Scores on the MoCA less than _____ are generally considered as abnormal.   26

One advantage of performing the MoCA test is that it includes a clock-drawing task.

One advantage of performing the MoCA test is that it includes a _____-drawing task.   clock-

Clock-drawing enables the examiner to assess the patient's ability to organize and to plan the placement of numbers on the clock.

Clock-drawing enables the examiner to assess the patient's ability to organize and to plan the placement of _____ on the clock.   numbers

Poor planning and irregular spacing between the numbers might indicate frontal lobe or executive dysfunction.

Poor planning and irregular spacing between the numbers might indicate frontal lobe or _____ dysfunction.

executive

Another screening test for cognitive dysfunction is the Confusion Assessment Method for the ICU, abbreviated CAM-ICU.

Another _____ test for cognitive dysfunction is the _____ _____ _____ for the ICU, abbreviated CAM-ICU.

screening

Confusion; Assessment; Method

The CAM-ICU can be administered in several minutes by physicians or nurses with minimal training and with a high degree of reliability, sensitivity, and specificity.

The CAM-ICU can be administered in several minutes by physicians or nurses with minimal _____ and with a high degree of reliability, sensitivity, and specificity.

training

The CAM-ICU is organized into several different categories, including historical features (e.g., acute onset or fluctuating course), attention and concentration ability, thinking (e.g., organized or disorganized), and level of consciousness.

The CAM-ICU is organized into several different categories, including historical features (e.g., _____ onset or fluctuating course), attention and _____ ability, thinking (e.g., organized or disorganized), and level of _____.

acute

concentration

consciousness

Acute changes in behavior or mental status require rapid recognition and treatment.

Acute changes in behavior or mental status require rapid recognition and _____.

treatment

Patients who are agitated and confused can be restless and disorganized or have illusions, hallucinations, delusions, or paranoid ideation.

Patients who are agitated and confused can be restless and disorganized or have illusions, _____, delusions, or paranoid ideation.

hallucinations

Agitation is manifest by excessive, usually non-purposeful, motor activity and internal tension.

_____ is manifest by excessive, usually non-purposeful, motor activity and internal tension.

Agitation

Agitation can vary in intensity from a state of mild restlessness to one of violent combativeness.

Agitation can vary in intensity from a state of mild _____ to one of violent combativeness.

restlessness

High degrees of agitation can jeopardize a patient's health (e.g., by compromising the patient's cardiovascular system).

High degrees of _____ can jeopardize a patient's health (e.g., by compromising the patient's cardiovascular system).

agitation

If left untreated, agitation can jeopardize the safety of the patient and the staff.

If left untreated, agitation can jeopardize the safety of the patient and the _____.

staff

At the very least, agitation can be a nuisance to staff and sap their emotional and physical resources.

At the very least, agitation can be a nuisance to _____ *and sap their emotional and physical resources.*

staff

Patients who are agitated and confused might be restless and have delusions, hallucinations, and paranoid ideation.

Patients who are agitated and confused might be restless and have delusions, _____, *and paranoid ideation.*

hallucinations

The confused patient is often restless or disorganized.

The confused patient is often restless or _____.

disorganized

Illusions, hallucinations, and paranoia are common in patients with an altered mental status and can precipitate agitation and combativeness.

Illusions, hallucinations, and paranoia are common in patients with an altered _____ _____ *and can precipitate agitation and combativeness.*

mental; status

An illusion is a misperception of reality that can affect any sensory modality; it can be visual, auditory, tactile, gustatory, or olfactory.

An _____ is a misperception of reality that can affect any sensory modality; it can be visual, auditory, tactile, gustatory, or olfactory.

illusion

If a man has a Foley catheter taped to his leg and says that he sees a snake crawling over his leg, he is likely having an illusion.

If a man has a Foley catheter taped to his leg and says that he sees a snake crawling over his leg, he is likely having an _____.

illusion

A hallucination is also a misperception of reality; however, a hallucination "makes something out of nothing."

A hallucination is also a misperception of _____; however, a hallucination "makes something out of nothing."

reality

If a man has nothing in or on his hand and says that he is holding a cigar, he is having a hallucination.

If a man has nothing in or on his hand and says that he is holding a cigar, he is having a _____.

hallucination

Hallucinations might involve hearing things that others don't hear, seeing things that aren't there, feeling things crawling on or under one's skin when there is nothing there, smelling things that aren't there, or tasting things without having something in one's mouth.

_____ might involve hearing things that others don't _____, seeing things that aren't there, feeling things crawling on or under one's skin when there is nothing there, smelling things that aren't there, or tasting things without having something in one's _____.

Hallucinations
hear

mouth

Hallucinations can involve any of the five senses.

Hallucinations can involve any of the five _____

senses

Paranoia is the false feeling or belief that someone is trying to deceive, harm, follow, or kill you.

Paranoia is the false feeling or _____ that someone is trying to deceive, _____, follow, or kill you.

belief
harm

The false belief that doctors and nurses are trying to hurt you is called paranoia or a paranoid delusion.

The false belief that doctors and nurses are trying to hurt you is called _____ or a paranoid delusion.

paranoia

When one has a fixed, false belief, it is called a delusion.

When one has a fixed, false belief, it is called a _____.

delusion

If you believe that you have heard your doctors and nurses plotting your demise while conferring outside your room, you are probably experiencing a paranoid delusion.

If you believe that you have heard your doctors and nurses plotting your demise while conferring outside your room, you are probably experiencing a _____ delusion.

The first steps in the appropriate management of agitation involve assuring the safety of the patient and the staff.

The first steps in the appropriate management of agitation involve assuring the _____ of the patient and the staff.

safety

Because management is predicated on etiology, it is crucial to evaluate the underlying cause of agitation and an altered mental status.

Because management is predicated on _____, it is crucial to evaluate the underlying cause of agitation and an altered mental status.

etiology

Agitation is not a specific diagnosis.

Agitation is not a specific _____.

diagnosis

Agitation is a behavioral manifestation that has many causes.

Agitation is a syndrome having many _____ or causes.

etiologies

Proper identification of the causes of agitation is important so that specific treatment can be administered.

Proper _____ *of the causes of agitation is important so that specific treatment can be administered.*

identification

Treatment with the appropriate agent or correction of the underlying medical or metabolic abnormalities will lead to more rapid resolution of the problem.

Treatment with the appropriate agent or correction of the underlying medical or metabolic _____ *will lead to more rapid resolution of the problem.*

abnormalities

Many factors contribute to the development of agitation.

Many factors contribute to the development of _____ .

agitation

Factors that predispose to agitation and delirium include the presence of serious medical illness, a history of central nervous system dysfunction, a history of psychiatric illness, and a personality type that limits an individual's coping ability.

Factors that predispose to agitation and delirium include the presence of serious medical illness, a history of _____ _____ _____ *dysfunction, a history of psychiatric illness, and a personality type that limits an individual's coping ability.*

central; nervous; system

Unfortunately, patients with agitation and or delirium are often thought to suffer from ICU psychosis.

Unfortunately, patients with agitation and or delirium are often thought to suffer from ICU _____.

psychosis

However, the term ICU psychosis is a misleading term.

However, the term ICU _____ *is a misleading term.*

psychosis

The term "ICU psychosis" implies to many practitioners that being in an ICU causes one to be psychotic, agitated, or confused.

*The term "*_____*" implies to many practitioners that being in an ICU causes one to be psychotic, agitated, or confused.*

ICU psychosis

Rarely does the stress associated with intensive care lead to a psychotic state.

Rarely does the stress associated with intensive care lead to a _____ *state.*

psychotic

The term "ICU psychosis" implies a cause-and-effect relationship between being in an ICU and becoming psychotic or agitated.

*The term "*_____*" implies a cause-and-effect relationship between being in an ICU and becoming psychotic or agitated.*

ICU psychosis

By way of comparison, cardiac arrhythmias often develop in critically ill individuals, but intensivists rarely, if ever, blame the ICU environment for these arrhythmias.

By way of comparison, cardiac _____ often develop in critically ill individuals, but intensivists rarely, if ever, blame the _____ environment for these arrhythmias.

arrhythmias

ICU

Some practitioners have maintained that a transfer out of the ICU is the appropriate treatment for the agitated and confused patient.

Some practitioners have maintained that a transfer out of the _____ is the appropriate treatment for the agitated and confused patient.

ICU

Unfortunately, transfer of an agitated patient to a lower level of care is, in general, not in the best interest of the patient.

Unfortunately, _____ of an agitated patient to a lower level of care is, in general, not in the best interest of the patient.

transfer

Few cardiologists would transfer a patient with a ventricular arrhythmia out of the ICU because he or she believed the ICU environment caused the arrhythmia.

Few cardiologists would transfer a patient with a ventricular _____ out of the ICU because he or she believed the ICU environment caused the arrhythmia.

arrhythmia

When a patient is agitated or psychotic in the ICU, a search for potential causes must be undertaken.

When a patient is agitated or psychotic in the ICU, a search for potential _____ *must be undertaken.*   causes

Psychosis is a syndrome involving a break from reality; it can occur when a patient is agitated or delirious.

Psychosis is a syndrome involving a break from _____*; it can occur when a patient is agitated or delirious.*   reality

Psychosis must be distinguished from agitation or delirium.

Psychosis must be distinguished from agitation or _____.   delirium

Psychosis must be distinguished from agitation or delirium to ensure that specific and appropriate treatment can be administered in a timely fashion.

Psychosis must be distinguished from agitation or delirium to ensure that specific and appropriate treatment can be administered in a _____ *fashion.*   timely

Psychosis is a loss of contact with reality.

Psychosis is a loss of contact with _____.   reality

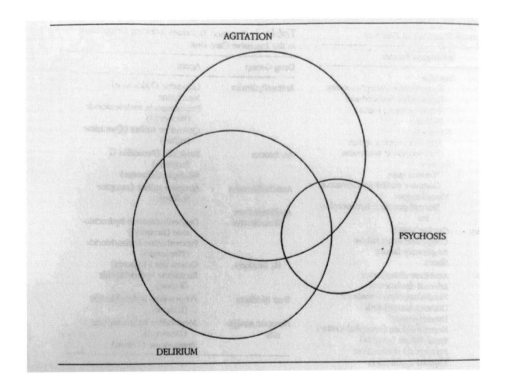

In psychiatric nomenclature, psychosis is generally considered to be idiopathic or functional (i.e., without an obvious organic etiology).

In psychiatric nomenclature, psychosis is generally considered to be _____ or functional (i.e., without an obvious organic etiology).

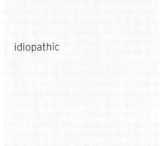

In most primary psychotic illnesses, thought process is abnormal and delusions and/or hallucinations often arise in the context of a normal sensorium.

In most primary psychotic illnesses, thought process is abnormal and delusions and/or _____ often arise in the context of a normal _____.

hallucinations
sensorium

Systematic delusions (i.e., with fixed, false beliefs) can occur in either psychosis or delirium.

Systematic delusions (i.e., with fixed, false _____) can occur in either psychosis or delirium.

beliefs

Idiopathic or primary psychotic illnesses include schizophrenia and bipolar disorder.

Idiopathic or primary psychotic illnesses include schizophrenia and _____ disorder.

bipolar

However, psychoses that develop in patients during a serious medical and neurological illness are rarely due to a primary psychotic illness.

However, _____ that develop in patients during a serious medical and neurological illness are rarely due to a primary psychotic illness.

psychoses

At times, a patient might be so severely agitated that he or she won't or can't cooperate with cognitive testing for assessment of orientation.

At times, a patient might be so severely agitated that he or she won't or can't _____ with cognitive testing for assessment of orientation.

cooperate

Under such circumstances, it is reasonable to assume that delirium or psychosis exists so that life-threatening conditions can be ruled-out and treated rapidly.

Under such circumstances, it is reasonable to assume that delirium or psychosis exists so that life-_____ conditions can be ruled-out and treated rapidly.

threatening

Delirium is a reversible organic condition that can result from severe medical illness.

Delirium is a _____ organic condition that can result from severe medical illness.

reversible

Typically, delirium is manifest by impairment of short-term memory, arousal, attention, the sleep–wake cycle, as well as by disorientation, perceptual abnormalities (e.g., illusions and hallucinations), and inappropriate behavior.

Typically, delirium is manifest by impairment of _____-_____ memory, arousal, attention, the sleep–wake cycle, as well as by disorientation, percep-tual abnormalities (e.g., _____, _____), and inappropriate behavior.

short-term

illusions; hallucinations

The mental status of the delirious patient fluctuates over a period of minutes to hours.

The mental status of the delirious patient_____ over a period of minutes to hours.

fluctuates

Have you heard the story about the two truck driv-ers? The driver didn't think that his directional signals were working, so he asked his buddy to get out of the truck to see if they were working. While looking at the signals his buddy said, "They're working, they're not working, they're working, they're not working, ..." That is the nature of delirium; it comes and goes.

One can see an agitated or confused patient at one moment and then a short while later see that person acting normally and think that everything is _____. One should be cautious about saying that a patient is not delirious after a single examination, because that individual might be having a lucid interval.

normal

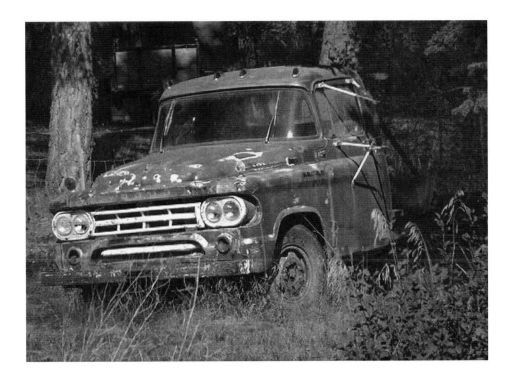

Hypervigilance and agitation are common in delirium, but psychomotor retardation can also be a feature of delirium.

Hypervigilance and _____ are common in delirium, but psychomotor retardation can also be a feature of delirium.

A delirious patient with psychomotor retardation is said to have hypoactive delirium.

_____ delirium is the label given to a delirious patient with psychomotor retardation.

Not uncommonly, a delirious patient will be uncooperative and refuse to answer questions; this limits our assessment of his or her mental status and forces us to rely more on our behavioral observations than on cognitive responses.

Not uncommonly, a delirious patient will be uncooperative and _____ to answer questions; this limits our assessment of his or her _____ status and forces us to rely more on our behavioral observations than on cognitive responses.

One must consider the diagnosis of delirium when patients are uncooperative because some patients attempt to cover up their cognitive impairment by not responding to the interviewer's questions.

One must consider the diagnosis of delirium when patients are _____ because some patients attempt to cover up their _____ impairment by not responding to the interviewer's questions.

Cognitive and behavioral abnormalities associated with delirium are often more apparent at night.

Cognitive and _____ abnormalities associated with delirium are often more apparent at _____.

behavioral

night

Delirious patients can be lucid and cooperative at one moment, and restless, agitated, disoriented, and confused the next.

Delirious patients can be _____ and cooperative at one moment, and restless, agitated, disoriented, and confused the next.

lucid

The diagnosis of delirium hinges on taking a careful history and performing a targeted physical examination, with a focus on potential etiologic factors.

The diagnosis of delirium hinges on taking a careful history and performing a targeted physical _____, with a focus on potential _____ factors.

examination
etiologic

The delirious patient is often restless and picks aimlessly at the bedsheets.

The delirious patient is often _____ and picks aimlessly at the bedsheets.

restless

Disorientation is typically present, but lucid intervals might occur in patients suffering from delirium.

Disorientation is _____ present, but _____ intervals might occur in patients suffering from delirium.

typically
lucid

Some patients attempt to cover up cognitive dysfunction by being uncooperative with the examination.

Some patients attempt to cover up _____ dysfunction by being _____ with the examination.

cognitive
uncooperative

Behavioral symptoms of mania (e.g., hyperactivity, rapid and loud talking, distractibility, decreased sleep, grandiosity, irritability, paranoia) might be seen in primary psychotic illnesses or in delirium (as caused by a toxic-metabolic disturbance).

Behavioral symptoms of _____ (e.g., hyperactivity, rapid and loud talking, distractibility, decreased sleep, grandiosity, irritability, paranoia) might be seen in primary psychotic illnesses or in delirium (as caused by a _____-_____ disturbance).

mania

toxic-metabolic

Symptoms of mania can be recalled by the mnemonic, DTR HIGH (deter the high), with each letter indicating a different symptom of mania (Distractibility, Talkativeness, Reckless behavior, Hyperactivity, Ideas that race, Grandiosity, and Hypersexuality). Three of these symptoms (with euphoria) for one week, or four of these symptoms (with irritability) for one week, qualifies for mania.

Symptoms of mania can be recalled by the mnemonic, _____ _____ (deter the high), with each letter indicating a different symptom of mania (Distractibility, Talkativeness, Reckless behavior, Hyperactivity, Ideas that race, Grandiosity, and Hypersexuality). Three of these symptoms (with _____) for one week, or four of these symptoms (with _____) for one week, qualifies for mania.

DTR; HIGH

euphoria
irritability

The presence of mania in a critically ill patient warrants a search for a toxic-metabolic organic disturbance.

The presence of _____ in a critically ill patient warrants a search for a toxic-metabolic organic disturbance.

mania

Drugs that are commonly associated with the development of mania include corticosteroids, isoniazid, and levodopa.

Drugs that are commonly associated with the development of mania include _____, isoniazid, and levodopa.

corticosteroids

Other secondary causes of mania include metabolic disturbances, infections, central nervous system neoplasms, and seizures (especially those that originate in the right temporal lobe).

Other secondary causes of mania include metabolic disturbances, infections, central nervous system neoplasms, and _____ (especially those that originate in the right temporal lobe).

seizures

High doses of corticosteroids (i.e., >80 mg/day of prednisone or its equivalent) might precipitate a manic syndrome.

High doses of corticosteroids (i.e., >80 mg/day of prednisone or its equivalent) might precipitate a _____ syndrome.

manic

When either delirium or psychosis occurs, an extensive differential diagnosis must be entertained.

When either delirium or psychosis occurs, an extensive _____ diagnosis must be entertained.

differential

Life-threatening causes of delirium can be recalled using the mnemonic, WWHHHHIIMMPS, with each letter of the mnemonic pertaining to one of the life-threatening causes.

Life-threatening _____ of delirium can be recalled using the _____, WWHHHHIIMMPS, with each letter of the mnemonic pertaining to one of the life-threatening causes.

causes
mnemonic

If left untreated, each of these causes can result in death.

If left _____, each of these causes can result in death.

untreated

The letter "W" in the mnemonic WWHHHHIIMMPS refers to Wernicke's encephalopathy, and withdrawal syndromes.

The letter "W" in the mnemonic WWHHHHIIMMPS refers to _____ encephalopathy, and withdrawal syndromes.

Wernicke's

Wernicke's encephalopathy can be rapidly diagnosed by the presence of ataxia, confusion, and ophthalmoplegia (or nystagmus).

_____ encephalopathy can be rapidly diagnosed by the presence of _____, confusion, and ophthalmoplegia (or nystagmus).

Wernicke's
ataxia

If ataxia, confusion, and ophthalmoplegia are observed, the diagnosis of Wernicke's encephalopathy should be considered and treatment with thiamine initiated, before glucose is administered.

If ataxia, confusion, and _____ are observed, the diagnosis of _____ encephalopathy should be considered and treatment with _____ initiated, before _____ is administered.

ophthalmoplegia
Wernicke's
thiamine
glucose

Serious withdrawal syndromes (reflecting one of the "W's" in the mnemonic) are those that work at the alcohol, benzodiazepine, and barbiturate receptor, and that have a pharmacological half-life of between 10 and 20 hours.

Serious withdrawal syndromes (reflecting one of the "W's" in the mnemonic) are those that that work at the alcohol, _____, and barbiturate receptor, and that have a pharmacological half-life of between _____ and _____ hours.

benzodiazepine

10; 20

The "H's" is in the mnemonic WWHHHHIIMMPS stand for hypoxia, hypoperfusion of the CNS, hypoglycemia, and hypertensive encephalopathy.

The "H's" is in the mnemonic WWHHHHIIMMPS stand for _____, hypoperfusion of the CNS, _____, and _____ encephalopathy.

hypoxia
hypoglycemia; hypertensive

Hypoxia should be considered if the patient is cyanotic, tachypneic, short of breath, and tachycardic.

_____ should be considered if the patient is cyanotic, tachypneic, short of breath, and tachycardic.

Hypoxia

Hypoxia can be confirmed by obtaining an oxygen saturation level or by determination of an arterial blood gas.

Hypoxia can be confirmed by obtaining an oxygen _____ level or by determination of an arterial blood gas.

saturation

Conditions that adversely affect cardiopulmonary function, such as congestive heart failure (CHF), pneumonia, or pulmonary embolism, increase the likelihood that one might become hypoxic and delirious.

Conditions that adversely affect cardiopulmonary function, such as congestive _____ _____ (CHF), pneumonia, or pulmonary _____, increase the likelihood that one might become _____ and delirious.

heart
failure
embolism
hypoxic

Hypoglycemia is another life-threatening cause of delirium that starts with the letter "H."

Hypoglycemia is another life-threatening cause of _____ that starts with the letter "H."

delirium

Delirium secondary to hypoglycemia is manifest by symptoms consistent with adrenergic excess.

Delirium secondary to hypoglycemia is manifest by symptoms consistent with _____ excess.

adrenergic

Symptoms consistent with adrenergic excess often occur in those afflicted by diabetes.

Symptoms consistent with adrenergic excess often occur in those afflicted by _____.

diabetes

Hypoglycemia is typically manifest by moist skin, mydriasis, and tachycardia, as well as by symptoms of CNS disturbance.

Hypoglycemia is typically manifest by _____ skin, _____, and _____, as well as by symptoms of a CNS disturbance.

moist

mydriasis; tachycardia

Delirium with adrenergic-mediated delirium—as can be caused by hypoglycemia—can be differentiated from anticholinergic-induced delirium (e.g., as might be caused by administration of atropine) because the skin is moist with hypoglycemia and dry with anticholinergic delirium.

Delirium with adrenergic-mediated delirium—as can be caused by hypoglycemia—can be differentiated from _____-induced delirium (e.g., as might be caused by administration of atropine) because the skin is moist with hypoglycemia and _____ with anticholinergic delirium.

anticholinergic-

dry

Treatment of hypoglycemia-induced delirium can be successfully achieved with an infusion of glucose (e.g., 50 mL of the D50 solution).

Treatment of hypoglycemia-induced delirium can be successfully achieved with an infusion of_____ (e.g., 50 mL of the D50 solution).

glucose

The third "H" in the mnemonic, WWHHHHIIMMPS, stands for hypertensive encephalopathy.

The third "H" in the mnemonic, WWHHHHIIMMPS, stands for _____ encephalopathy.

hypertensive

The fastest method for detecting hypertensive encephalopathy is to check the blood pressure.

The fastest method for detecting hypertensive enceph-alopathy is to check the blood _____.

pressure

If the blood pressure is very high, use of antihypertensive agents is appropriate.

If the blood pressure is very _____, use of _____ agents is appropriate.

high
antihypertensive

Funduscopic examination of the patient might be nearly impossible with an agitated hypertensive patient because of his or her inability to cooperate with the exam.

_____ examination of the patient might be nearly impossible with an agitated hypertensive patient because of his or her inability to cooperate with the exam.

Funduscopic

Funduscopic examination of an agitated hypertensive patient can be dangerous for the examiner because the examiner's ophthalmoscope could be thrust into his or her own eye.

Funduscopic examination of an agitated hypertensive patient can be dangerous for the examiner because the examiner's _____ could be thrust into his or her own eye.

ophthalmoscope

The "I's" in the mnemonic WWHHHHIIMMPS stands for intracerebral hemorrhage and infection.

The "I's" in the mnemonic WWHHHHIIMMPS stands for _____ _____ and _____.

intracerebral; hemorrhage;
infection

Symptoms of intracerebral hemorrhage include headache and photophobia, and there might also be evidence of CNS trauma.

Symptoms of intracerebral hemorrhage include _____ and _____, and there might also be evidence of CNS trauma.

headache; photophobia

A history of head trauma or observation of battle signs (periauricular ecchymosis) or raccoon signs (periorbital ecchymosis) should suggest a diagnosis of intracerebral hemorrhage.

A history of head trauma or observation of _____ _____ (periauricular ecchymosis) or _____ _____ (periorbital ecchymosis) should suggest a diagnosis of intracerebral hemorrhage.

battle; signs
raccoon; signs

A computerized tomographic (CT) scan or magnetic resonance imaging (MRI) study of the head will confirm the diagnosis of an intracerebral hemorrhage.

A computerized tomographic (CT) scan or magnetic resonance imaging (MRI) study of the head will confirm the diagnosis of an _____ _____.

intracerebral; hemorrhage

Xanthochromia, caused by having red blood cells present in the cerebrospinal fluid (CSF) should also heighten one's suspicion that an intracerebral hemorrhage has occurred.

_____, caused by having red blood cells present in the _____ _____ (CSF) should also heighten one's suspicion that an _____ hemorrhage has occurred.

Xanthochromia
cerebrospinal; fluid
intracerebral

The "M's" in the mnemonic, WWHHHHIIMMPS, stands for meningitis and metabolic derangement.

The "M's" in the mnemonic, WWHHHHIIMMPS, stands for _____ and _____ derangement.

meningitis; metabolic

Meningitis and encephalitis are life-threatening causes of delirium that can present with an abnormal mental status.

Meningitis and _____ are life-threatening causes of delirium that can present with an abnormal mental status.

encephalitis

Headache, fever, and an elevated white blood cell (WBC) count, as well as nuchal rigidity are suggestive of meningitis.

Headache, fever, and an elevated _____ _____ _____ (WBC) count, as well as _____ rigidity are suggestive of meningitis.

white
blood; cell
nuchal

Confirmation of the diagnosis of meningitis can be obtained by finding white blood cells (WBCs) in the CSF.

Confirmation of the diagnosis of _____ can be obtained by finding white blood cells (WBCs) in the CSF.

meningitis

However, in immunocompromised patients and in the elderly, fever and an elevated WBC count might not always be present.

However, in _____ patients and in the elderly, fever and an elevated WBC count might not always be present.

immunocompromised

Immunocompromised patients—for example, those with acquired immunodeficiency syndrome [AIDS]—are at higher risk for the sudden development of meningitis and central nervous system (CNS) tumors that can adversely alter an individual's mental status.

Immunocompromised patients—for example, those with acquired immunodeficiency syndrome [AIDS]—are at higher risk for the sudden development of _____ and CNS tumors that can adversely alter an individual's _____ status.

meningitis
mental

After the diagnosis of meningitis or encephalitis has been made, appropriate treatment with antibiotics or antiviral agents should be initiated.

After the diagnosis of meningitis or encephalitis has been made, appropriate treatment with antibiotics or antiviral agents should be _____.

initiated

The "P" in the mnemonic WWHHHHIIMMPS is for poisoning.

The "P" in the mnemonic WWHHHHIIMMPS is for _____.

poisoning

Not uncommonly, drug-induced delirium can result from administration of excessive amounts of atropine or other anticholinergic agents (e.g., tricyclic antidepressants).

Not uncommonly, drug-induced delirium can result from administration of excessive amounts of atropine or other _____ agents (e.g., tricyclic antidepressants).

anticholinergic

An assortment of signs and symptoms (e.g., confusion, mydriasis, tachycardia, red and dry skin, as well as reduced bowel sounds) are often found in patients with anticholinergic delirium.

An assortment of signs and _____ (e.g., _____, _____, _____, _____ and _____ skin, as well as reduced _____ sounds) are often found in patients with anticholinergic excess.

symptoms; confusion
mydriasis; tachycardia; red
dry; bowel

Although most practitioners are conservative and wait for the metabolism and clearance of anticholinergic excess, others attempt to reverse the syndrome by administration of the antidote, physostigmine.

Although most practitioners are conservative and wait for the metabolism and clearance of anticholinergic excess, others attempt to reverse the syndrome by administration of the _____, physostigmine.

antidote

Physostigmine has been used safely to diagnose and to treat (or reverse) anticholinergic delirium via a slow intravenous infusion.

_____ has been used safely to diagnose and to treat (or reverse) _____ delirium via a slowly administered intravenous infusion.

Physostigmine
anticholinergic

A continuous infusion of physostigmine has been used to treat an extremely agitated patient with anticholinergic delirium.

A continuous infusion of _____ has been used to treat an extremely agitated patient with anticholinergic delirium.

physostigmine

One way to remember the signs and symptoms of anticholinergic delirium is to think of the saying:

Mad as a hatter: to recall the confusion associated with this condition;

Blind as a bat: to recall the pupillary dilatation with anticholinergic excess;

Hot as a hare: to recall the presence of fever;

Red as a beet: to recall the flushed skin;

Dry as a bone: to recall the dry skin; and,

Plugged as a pump: to recall urinary retention and ileus associated with anticholinergic delirium.

One way to remember the signs and symptoms of anticholinergic delirium is to think of the saying:

_____ as a hatter: to recall the _____ associated with this condition;   Mad; confusion

_____ as a bat: to recall the _____ _____ with anticholinergic excess;   Blind; pupillary dilatation

_____ as a hare: to recall the presence of _____;   Hot / fever

_____ as a beet: to recall the _____ skin;   Red; flushed

_____ as a bone; and,   Dry

_____ as a pump: to recall _____ retention and _____ associated with anticholinergic delirium.   Plugged; urinary ileus

The "S" in the mnemonic WWHHHHIIMMPS" stands for seizures.

The "S" in the mnemonic WWHHHHIIMMPS" stands for _____.   seizures

After you consider the life-threatening causes of delirium (by using the mnemonic WWHHHHIIMMPS) you should continue to search for other causes of delirium.

After you consider the life-threatening causes of _____ (by using the mnemonic _____) you should continue to search for other causes of delirium.

delirium; WWHHHHIIMMPS

Delirium has been attributed to dysfunction of the CNS, the cardiopulmonary system, and the endocrine system. In addition, metabolic abnormalities, infections, intoxication or withdrawal from centrally-acting agents, nutritional deficiencies, and poisons, can cause delirium.

Delirium has been attributed to dysfunction of the _____, the cardiopulmonary system, and the endocrine system. In addition, metabolic abnormalities, infections, intoxication or _____ from centrally-acting agents, nutritional deficiencies, and poisons, can cause _____.

CNS

withdrawal

delirium

Conditions known to cause CNS dysfunction can be categorized as vascular (e.g., hypertensive encephalopathy, intracerebral hemorrhage, vasculitis, and stroke), neoplastic (e.g., secondary to a space-occupying lesion, or a paraneoplastic syndrome), seizure-related (e.g., a post-ictal state or complex partial seizures), or miscellaneous conditions (e.g., normal pressure hydrocephalus [NPH]).

Conditions known to cause CNS dysfunction can be categorized as vascular (e.g., hypertensive _____, intracerebral _____, vasculitis, and stroke), neoplastic (e.g., secondary to a space-_____ lesion, or a _____ syndrome), seizure-related (e.g., a post-ictal state or complex partial seizures), or miscellaneous conditions (e.g., normal _____ hydrocephalus [NPH]).

encephalopathy
hemorrhage
occupying
paraneoplastic

pressure

Therefore, several categories of CNS dysfunction (e.g., vascular, neoplastic, and seizure-related conditions) should be reviewed when evaluating a delirious patient.

Therefore, several categories for CNS _____ (e.g., vascular, _____, and seizure-related conditions) should be reviewed when evaluating a delirious patient.

dysfunction
neoplastic

Cardiopulmonary dysfunction can also cause delirium.

Cardiopulmonary dysfunction can also cause _____.

delirium

Cardiopulmonary causes of delirium include: cardiac arrest, congestive heart failure (CHF), respiratory failure, and shock.

Cardiopulmonary causes of delirium include: cardiac _____, congestive _____ _____ (CHF), respiratory _____, and _____.

arrest; heart
failure; failure
shock

If cardiac arrest, heart failure, or shock go untreated, delirium might not be the patient's biggest problem, as death might ensue.

If cardiac arrest, heart failure, or shock go untreated, delirium might not be the patient's biggest problem, as _____ might ensue.

death

Correction of the underlying cardiopulmonary process is required before delirium will be successfully treated.

Correction of the underlying cardiopulmonary process is required before delirium will be successfully _____.

treated

Endocrine and metabolic abnormalities include acid-base disturbances, adrenal dysfunction, fluid and electrolyte imbalance, diabetic ketoacidosis, hypoglycemia, hepatic failure, parathyroid dysfunction, and porphyria.

Endocrine and _____ abnormalities include acid-base disturbances, adrenal dysfunction, fluid and electrolyte imbalance, diabetic ketoacidosis, hypoglycemia, hepatic failure, parathyroid dysfunction, and porphyria.

metabolic

Hyponatremia, hypoglycemia, and hepatic failure are among the more common endocrine and metabolic abnormalities that lead to delirium.

Hyponatremia, hypoglycemia, and hepatic failure are among the more common _____ and metabolic abnormalities that lead to delirium.

endocrine

Meningitis, encephalitis, sepsis, sub-acute bacterial endocarditis, and tertiary syphilis are infection-related causes of delirium.

Meningitis, _____, *sepsis,* *sub-acute* _____ *endocarditis, and tertiary* _____ *are infection-related causes of delirium.*

encephalitis
bacterial; syphilis

Intoxication or withdrawal from a variety of agents can lead to delirium.

Intoxication or _____ *from a variety of agents can lead to delirium.*

withdrawal

Excessive use of or withdrawal from anesthetics, anticholinergic agents, hallucinogens, psychostimulants (e.g., amphetamines, cocaine), narcotics, and sedative-hypnotic drugs (e.g., barbiturates, benzodiazepines) can cause delirium.

Excessive use of or withdrawal from anesthetics, anticholinergic agents, hallucinogens, psychostimulants (e.g., _____, _____), *narcotics, and sedative-* _____ *drugs (e.g., barbiturates,* _____*) can cause delirium.*

amphetamines; cocaine
hypnotic
benzodiazepines

Withdrawal reactions from alcohol and sedative-hypnotic agents are more common as a cause of delirium than are withdrawal from psychostimulants, or from narcotics.

Withdrawal reactions from alcohol and _____- *hypnotic agents are more common as a cause of delirium than are withdrawal from psychostimulants, or from* _____*.*

sedative-

narcotics

Deficiencies in folic acid, niacin, thiamine, and vitamin B_{12} are examples of nutritional deficiencies that lead to delirium.

Deficiencies in folic _____, *niacin,* _____, *and vitamin B_{12} are examples of nutritional* _____ *that lead to delirium.*

acid
thiamine
deficiencies

Niacin deficiency leads to pellagra, thiamine deficiency leads to Wernicke's encephalopathy and to Wernicke-Korsakoff psychosis, whereas vitamin B_{12} deficiency leads to pernicious anemia.

Niacin deficiency leads to _____, *thiamine deficiency leads to* _____ *encephalopathy and to Wernicke-*_____ *psychosis, whereas vitamin B_{12} deficiency leads to* _____ *anemia.*

pellagra
Wernicke's
Korsakoff
pernicious

The triad of ataxia, confusion, and ophthalmoplegia is characteristic of Wernicke's encephalopathy.

The triad of _____, _____, *and* _____ *is characteristic of Wernicke's encephalopathy.*

ataxia; confusion
ophthalmoplegia

When a patient is suspected of having Wernicke's encephalopathy, he or she should be treated promptly with thiamine, before infusion of glucose, so that the disorder can be reversed.

When a patient is suspected of having _____ *encephalopathy, he or she should be treated promptly with* _____, _____ *infusion of glucose, so that the disorder can be reversed.*

Wernicke's

thiamine; before

Poisoning with a variety of substances—for example, carbon monoxide, heavy metals (e.g., lead, manganese, mercury), and toxins—can lead to delirium.

_____ with a variety of substances—for example, carbon monoxide, heavy metals (e.g., lead, manganese, mercury), and toxins—can lead to _____.

Poisoning

delirium

Performing a toxic screen analysis can be useful in the detection of poisons (e.g., carbon monoxide, heavy metals, other toxins).

_Performing a _____ _____ analysis can be useful in the detection of _____ (e.g., carbon monoxide, heavy metals, other toxins)._

toxic; screen
poisons

Several classes of drugs commonly used in ICUs have been linked with causing delirium.

_Several classes of _____ commonly used in ICUs have been linked with causing delirium._

drugs

Drugs associated with delirium include antiarrhythmics, antibiotics, anticholinergics, antihistamines, beta-blockers, and narcotic analgesics.

_Drugs associated with delirium include: _____, antibiotics, _____, antihistamines, beta-blockers, and narcotic analgesics._

antiarrhythmics
anticholinergics

Antiarrhythmics, such as lidocaine, mexiletine, procainamide, and quinidine sulfate can cause delirium.

_____, such as lidocaine, mexiletine, procainamide, and quinidine sulfate can cause delirium._

Antiarrhythmics

At higher doses, antiarrhythmics can cause generalized or partial seizures.

At higher doses, _____ can cause generalized or partial _____.

antiarrhythmics
seizures

In general, the prevalence of mental status changes increases as the dose of the antiarrhythmic agent increases and the metabolism of the patient decreases.

In general, the prevalence of mental _____ changes increases as the dose of the antiarrhythmic agent _____ and the metabolism of the patient _____.

status

increases
decreases

Older patients on antiarrhythmic drugs frequently need to have the dose of their antiarrhythmic drug decreased to minimize mental status changes.

Older patients on antiarrhythmic drugs frequently need to have the dose of their antiarrhythmic drug _____ to minimize mental status changes.

decreased

Among antibiotics, penicillin, at high doses, has been associated with delirium.

Among antibiotics, _____, at high doses, has been associated with delirium.

penicillin

Atropine use might cause anticholinergic delirium and be accompanied by mydriasis, dry skin, tachycardia, urinary retention, and decreased bowel motility.

Atropine use might cause _____ delirium and be accompanied by mydriasis, dry _____, tachycardia, urinary _____, and decreased bowel motility.

anticholinergic
skin
retention

Diphenhydramine and promethazine are non-selective antihistamines associated with delirium.

Diphenhydramine and promethazine are non-selective _____ associated with delirium.

antihistamines

Cimetidine and ranitidine are histamine blockers associated with delirium.

Cimetidine and ranitidine are histamine _____ associated with delirium.

blockers

Doses of many delirium-inducing drugs need to be decreased as hepatic metabolism or renal function become impaired.

Doses of many delirium-_____ drugs need to be decreased as hepatic metabolism or renal function become impaired.

inducing

When renal function becomes impaired, the dose of cimetidine needs to be decreased to minimize or to avoid mental status changes from occurring.

When renal function becomes _____, the dose of cimetidine needs to be _____ to minimize or to avoid mental status changes from occurring.

Impaired
decreased

Among the narcotics, meperidine and pentazocin are the most likely to cause delirium.

Among the narcotics, _____ and _____ are the most likely to cause delirium.

meperidine; pentazocin

When parenteral meperidine is administered at doses greater than or equal to 300 mg per day for three days or more, normeperidine toxicity becomes common, appearing in one-third of those so treated.

When parenteral _____ is administered at doses greater than or equal to _____ mg per day for three days or more, normeperidine _____ becomes common, appearing in one-_____ of those so treated.

meperidine
300
toxicity
third

Delirium is an organic brain syndrome marked by a clouded state of consciousness, distractibility, decreased attention, sensory misperceptions, and a fluctuating course.

Delirium is an organic _____ _____ marked by a clouded state of _____, distractibility, decreased attention, sensory _____, and a fluctuating course.

brain; syndrome
consciousness
misperceptions

An alternative name for delirium might well be "acute brain failure"; this would serve to distinguish it from "chronic brain failure," or dementia.

An alternative name for delirium might well be "_____ brain failure"; this would serve to distinguish it from "_____ brain failure," or dementia.

acute
chronic

Although dementing illnesses can reveal perceptual disturbances, incoherent speech, disturbed sleep–wake cycles, increased or decreased activity, disorientation, and memory impairment, a fluctuating course is far more characteristic of delirium.

Although dementing illnesses can reveal perceptual disturbances, incoherent speech, disturbed sleep–wake cycles, increased or decreased activity, disorientation, and memory impairment, a fluctuating course is far more characteristic of _____.

delirium

Associated features of delirium include anxiety, fear, irritability, depression, euphoria, and apathy.

Associated features of delirium include anxiety, fear, _____, depression, euphoria, and _____.

irritability
apathy

Presence of affective features broadens the differential diagnosis, given that many individuals with delirium have comorbid conditions.

Presence of affective features broadens the differential diagnosis, given that many individuals with delirium have _____ conditions.

comorbid

It is crucial to remember that treatment of delirium is predicated on the etiology of delirium.

It is crucial to remember that treatment of delirium is predicated on the _____ of delirium.

etiology

Identification of the etiology of delirium facilitates initiation of the specific treatment for delirium.

Identification of the etiology of delirium facilitates initiation of the _____ treatment for delirium.

specific

If delirium is caused by hypoxemia, the treatment is oxygen, not an antipsychotic such as haloperidol.

If delirium is caused by hypoxemia, the treatment is _____, not an antipsychotic such as haloperidol.

oxygen

If delirium is caused by hypogylcemia, the treatment is glucose, not an antipsychotic such as haloperidol.

If delirium is caused by hypogylcemia, the treatment is _____, not an antipsychotic such as haloperidol.

glucose

You should always be prepared to consider and rule-out life-threatening causes of delirium.

You should always be prepared to consider and rule-out _____-_____ causes of delirium.

life-threatening

The treatment of an agitated and delirious patient involves correction of metabolic and systemic abnormalities, elimination of drug toxicity, removal of the offending agent(s), and administration of the appropriate antidote (such as physostigmine, naloxone, or flumazenil).

The treatment of an agitated and delirious patient involves correction of _____ _____, elimination of _____ _____, removal of the _____ _____, and administration of the appropriate _____ (such as physostigmine, naloxone, or flumazenil).

metabolic; abnormalities
drug; toxicity
offending; agent(s)
antidote(s)

Physostigmine reverses anticholinergic toxicity, naloxone reverses narcotic overdoses, and flumazenil reverses benzodiazepine overdoses.

Physostigmine reverses _____ toxicity, naloxone reverses _____ overdoses, and flumazenil reverses _____ overdoses.

anticholinergic
narcotic
benzodiazepine

You must remember that withdrawal from drugs that work at the alcohol, benzodiazepine, and barbiturate receptor can all lead to withdrawal syndromes.

You must remember that withdrawal from drugs that work at the alcohol, benzodiazepine, and barbiturate receptor can all lead to _____ syndromes.

withdrawal

Drugs with a half-life of 10 to 20 hours have the most frequent and most intense withdrawal syndromes after sudden discontinuation or a dramatic decrease in the size of the administered dose.

Drugs with a half-life of _____ to _____ hours have the most frequent and most intense _____ syndromes after sudden _____ or a dramatic _____ in the size of the admin-istered dose.

10; 20

withdrawal; discontinuation
decrease

Withdrawal symptoms following discontinuation or a decrease in the narcotic dose are common but rarely severe enough to cause delirium.

Withdrawal symptoms following discontinuation or a decrease in the narcotic dose are common but rarely severe enough to cause _____.

delirium

Onset of withdrawal symptoms is a function of the half-life of the drug being used; the longer the half-life, the longer the time from taking the last dose to the development of the signs and symptoms of withdrawal.

Onset of withdrawal symptoms is a function of the _____-_____ of the drug being used; the longer the half-life, the longer the time from taking the last dose to the development of the signs and symp-toms of _____.

half-life

withdrawal

Withdrawal symptom frequency and intensity is greatest with drugs having a half-life of between 10 and 20 hours.

Withdrawal symptom frequency and intensity is greatest with drugs having a _____-_____ of between _____ and _____ hours.

Replacement of a drug with a drug having a longer half-life and that works at the same receptors manages withdrawal symptoms.

Replacement of a drug with a drug having a _____ half-life and that works at the same receptors manages withdrawal symptoms.

Clonidine, an alpha agonist, is effective in reducing the signs and symptoms of narcotic withdrawal.

Clonidine, an _____ agonist, is effective in reducing the signs and symptoms of _____ withdrawal.

Haloperidol is an effective agent for the signs and symptoms of delirium from many etiologies.

_____ is an effective agent for the signs and symptoms of delirium from many etiologies.

Haloperidol has trivial effects on heart rate, blood pressure, and respiratory drive.

Haloperidol has trivial effects on heart rate, blood _____, and respiratory drive.

Although intravenous (IV) haloperidol has never been approved by the Food and Drug Administration (FDA), it has been used widely across the country in ICUs.

Although _____ haloperidol has never been approved by the Food and Drug Administration (FDA), it has been used widely across the country in ICUs.

intravenous (IV)

Before using IV haloperidol, you should always flush the IV line with a saline solution because IV haloperidol precipitates with phenytoin and heparin.

Before using IV haloperidol, you should always flush the IV line with a saline solution because IV haloperidol precipitates with _____ and _____

phenytoin; heparin

The dose of IV haloperidol used to treat agitation depends largely on the severity of the symptoms.

The dose of IV haloperidol used to treat agitation depends largely on the _____ of the symptoms.

severity

The onset of action of IV haloperidol is between 10 and 30 minutes.

The onset of action of IV haloperidol is between _____ and _____ minutes.

10; 30

Hypotension is an uncommon side effect of IV haloperidol; when it occurs, it is most often associated with hypovolemia.

Hypotension is an uncommon side effect of IV haloperidol; when it occurs, it is most often associated with _____.

hypovolemia

Use of IV haloperidol can lead to QTc prolongation and torsades de pointes, a polymorphic ventricular tachycardia.

Use of IV haloperidol can lead to QTc _____ *and* _____ _____ _____, *a polymorphic ventricular tachycardia.*

prolongation
torsades; de; pointes

Extrapyramidal symptoms (EPS) from IV haloperidol are very uncommon; EPS are much more common after oral administration (15%) or after intramuscular use (40%).

Extrapyramidal symptoms (EPS) from IV haloperidol are very uncommon; EPS are much more common after _____ *administration (15%) or after* _____ *use (40%).*

oral
intramuscular

The dose of IV haloperidol is titrated to the severity of symptoms; if agitation is mild it is reasonable to start with 0.5 mg to 2 mg, if agitation is moderately severe it is reasonable to start with 5 mg to 10 mg, and if agitation is severe and is jeopardizing the safety of the patient or staff, it is reasonable to start with 10 mg, while being mindful of the QTc interval.

The dose of IV haloperidol is titrated to the _____ *of symptoms; if agitation is* _____ *it is reasonable to start with 0.5 mg to 2 mg, if agitation is moderately severe it is reasonable to start with* _____ *mg to* _____ *mg, and if agitation is* _____ *and is jeopardizing the safety of the patient or staff, it is reasonable to start with* _____ *mg, while being mindful of the QTc interval.*

severity
mild

5; 10
severe

10

The dose of IV haloperidol can be repeated every 15 to 30 minutes, or as necessary, and adjusted to the clinical course.

The dose of IV haloperidol can be repeated every _____ to _____ minutes, or as necessary, and adjusted to the clinical course.

15; 30

Monitoring of the QTc interval is appropriate during treatment with IV haloperidol.

Monitoring of the _____ interval is appropriate during treatment with IV haloperidol.

QTc

Antipsychotics, other than haloperidol, can also be used to treat agitated and delirious patients.

_____, other than haloperidol, can also be used to treat agitated and delirious patients.

Antipsychotics

Another antipsychotic, droperidol, is more sedating than haloperidol; it also lowers blood pressure more than does haloperidol.

Another antipsychotic, droperidol, is _____ sedating than haloperidol; it also lowers blood pressure _____ than does haloperidol.

more

more

Chlorpromazine, another antipsychotic agent, is more anticholinergic, more apt to induce hypotension, and more likely to induce arrhythmias than is haloperidol.

Chlorpromazine, another antipsychotic agent, is _____ anticholinergic, _____ apt to induce hypotension, and _____ likely to induce arrhythmias than is haloperidol.

more; more

more

Second-generation antipsychotics that can reduce agitation include olanzapine, quetiapine, risperidone, clozapine, and ziprasidone.

Second-generation antipsychotics that can reduce agitation include _____, _____, _____, _____, *and* _____.

olanzapine; quetiapine risperidone; clozapine; ziprasidone

Non-antipsychotic agents can also treat agitation; these include dexmedetomidine (a highly selective alpha-2 receptor agonist with analgesic properties), valproate (especially useful when irritability or impulsivity is present), propofol, narcotics, paralytics (which require co-administration of sedatives), and benzodiazepines (such as lorazepam or midazolam).

Non-antipsychotic agents can also treat agitation; these include _____ *(a highly selective alpha-2 receptor agonist with analgesic properties),* _____ *(especially useful when irritability or impulsivity is present), propofol,* _____, _____ *(which require co-administration of sedatives), and* _____ *(such as lorazepam or midazolam).*

dexmedetomidine

valproate
narcotics
paralytics
benzodiazepines

In addition, non-pharmacological treatments can help to reduce agitation.

In addition, non-_____ treatments can help to reduce agitation.

pharmacological

Non-pharmacological treatments of agitation include frequent reorientation, adjustments to the physical environment, reassurance, clarification of the patient's misconceptions, and appearing calm in the face of chaos and crisis.

Non-pharmacological treatments of agitation include frequent _____, adjustments to the _____ environment, _____, clarification of the patient's _____, and appearing _____ in the face of chaos and crisis.

reorientation; physical reassurance
misconceptions; calm

Even more important than treating delirium is the prevention of delirium.

Even more important than treating delirium is the _____ of delirium.

prevention

However, relatively few studies have been conducted to prevent delirium.

However, relatively few studies have been conducted to _____ delirium.

prevent

One strategy to prevent delirium is to reduce risk factors of delirium.

One strategy to prevent delirium is to reduce risk _____ of delirium.

factors

Optimizing oxygenation, assuring adequate levels of hemoglobin and blood pressure, and being mindful of risk factors for alcohol withdrawal can reduce the incidence of delirium.

Optimizing _____, assuring adequate _____ of hemoglobin and blood pressure, and being mindful of risk factors for alcohol _____ can reduce the incidence of delirium.

oxygenation
levels
withdrawal

You can also administer antipsychotics prophylactically to reduce the incidence of delirium.

You can also administer antipsychotics _____ to reduce the incidence of delirium.

prophylactically

In one study of postoperative delirium among elderly patients undergoing hip or knee replacement surgery, the incidence of post-operative delirium was reduced with administration of prophylactic doses (5 mg) of an atypical antipsychotic, olanzapine, given just before surgery and on arrival to the recovery room.

In one study of postoperative _____ among elderly patients undergoing hip or knee replacement surgery, the incidence of post-operative delirium was reduced with administration of _____ doses (5 g) of an atypical antipsychotic, _____, given just before surgery and on arrival to the recovery room.

delirium

prophylactic
olanzapine

In that study, the incidence of delirium was reduced from 41% to 15% and more patients could return home after hospital discharge.

In that study, the incidence of delirium was reduced from 41% to _____% and more patients could return home after hospital discharge.

15

Cognitive impairment is characteristic of both delirium and dementia.

Cognitive impairment is characteristic of both delirium and _____.

dementia

Dementia is a syndrome characterized by a clinically significant decline in memory as well as by at least one other area of higher cortical function.

Dementia is a syndrome characterized by a clinically significant decline in _____ as well as by at least one other area of higher _____ function.

memory
cortical

Dementia usually develops over months to years; this course differs from that of delirium, which has a more acute onset.

Dementia usually develops over _____ to _____; this course differs from that of delirium, which has a more acute _____.

months
years
onset

Dementia is linked to more than 80 different specific etiologies; some of these are common and others are rare.

Dementia is linked to more than 80 different specific etiologies; some of these are common and others are _____.

rare

Not all dementing illnesses are progressive.

Not all _____ illnesses are progressive.

dementing

Dementia is manifest by an acquired decline in memory.

Dementia is manifest by an acquired _____ in memory.

decline

Dementia is associated with an impairment in social or occupational functioning and by an impairment in at least one other area of higher cortical function.

Dementia is associated with an impairment in social or _____ functioning and by an impairment in at least one other area of _____ _____ function.

occupational
higher; cortical

Impairments in higher cortical function include aphasia, apraxia, agnosia, and executive dysfunction.

Impairments in higher cortical function include _____, _____, _____, and _____ _____.

aphasia; apraxia; agnosia
executive; dysfunction

Terminology needed to understand the components of cognitive impairment include aphasia (difficulty with language; e.g., speaking, reading, and repeating words), apraxia (an inability to carry out motor tasks despite intact motor function), agnosia (failure to recognize a familiar object despite intact sensory function), and executive dysfunction (involving problems with planning, abstraction, and sequencing).

Terminology needed to understand the components of cognitive impairment include: _____ (difficulty with language; e.g., speaking, reading, and repeating words), _____ (an inability to carry out motor tasks despite intact motor function), _____ (failure to recognize a familiar object despite intact sensory function), and _____ _____ (involving problems with planning, abstraction, and sequencing).

aphasia

apraxia
agnosia

executive; dysfunction

Dementia increases in frequency as age advances.

Dementia increases in frequency as _____   age
advances.

Roughly 15% of individuals older than 60 have a
dementing illness.

Roughly _____% of individuals older than 60   15
have a dementing illness.

The prevalence of dementia is 1% at age 60, and the
prevalence of dementia doubles every five years after
age 60; by age 85, the prevalence of dementia is 50%.

The prevalence of dementia is _____% at age   1
60, and the prevalence of dementia _____   doubles
every five years after age 60; by age 85, the prevalence
of dementia is _____%.   50

A familial pattern of transmission of dementia is found
in some conditions (e.g., Huntington's disease, which
has an autosomal dominant pattern).

A familial pattern of transmission of dementia is found
in some conditions (e.g., _____ disease, which   Huntington's
has an autosomal _____ pattern).   dominant

Early-onset Alzheimer's disease is associated with
several chromosomal mutations (e.g., homozygote
apolipoprotein E4 alleles).

Early-onset _____ disease is associated with   Alzheimer's
several chromosomal mutations (e.g., homozygote
_____ alleles).   apolipoprotein E4

Regarding the evaluation and treatment of patients with dementia, clinicians must remember that much can be done to help afflicted patients and their families. Even if the dementia is incurable, management can be facilitated.

Regarding the evaluation and treatment of patients with dementia, clinicians must remember that much can be done to help afflicted patients and their families. Even if the dementia is incurable, _____ can be facilitated.

management

When evaluating a patient with dementia, a complete history should be obtained, a medical and neurological examination conducted, and appropriate laboratory tests should be ordered.

When evaluating a patient with dementia, a complete _____ should be obtained, a medical and neurological _____ conducted, and appropriate _____ tests should be ordered.

history
examination
laboratory

The time course and description of symptoms and function of the patient with dementia is often best obtained from family members or friends because history obtained from the patient might be inaccurate or incomplete.

The time course and description of _____ and _____ of the patient with dementia is often best obtained from family members or friends because history obtained from the patient might be _____ or _____.

symptoms
function

inaccurate; incomplete

You should determine whether initial symptoms of dementia came on gradually or abruptly.

You should determine whether initial symptoms of dementia came on gradually or _____.

Dementia of the Alzheimer's type (DAT) and vascular dementia have different patterns of onset and course.

Dementia of the Alzheimer's type (DAT) and _____ dementia have different patterns of onset and course.

Disease progression is gradual with dementia of the Alzheimer's type, and stepwise with vascular dementia.

Disease progression is gradual with dementia of the _____ type, and stepwise with _____ dementia.

Clinicians should inquire about functional status and ask about how a patient with dementia spends his or her typical day at work and in leisure activities.

Clinicians should inquire about _____ status and ask about how a patient with dementia spends his or her typical day at work and in leisure activities.

Activities of daily living, and the need for assistance, should also be assessed; these activities include bathing, dressing, toileting, transferring, continence, and feeding.

Activities of _____ _____, *and the need for assistance, should also be assessed; these activities include* _____, _____, _____, _____, _____, *and* _____.

Instrumental activities of daily living involve performance of more complex tasks, such as ambulating, using the telephone, shopping, preparing meals, performing housework, doing laundry, self-administering medications, and managing money.

_____ *activities of daily living involve performance of more* _____ *tasks, such as* _____, _____, _____, _____, _____, _____, _____, _____, _____, *and* _____ _____ _____.

The clinical characteristics of Alzheimer's disease include an insidious onset of symptoms (e.g., memory deficits, verbal and spatial impairment).

The clinical characteristics of Alzheimer's disease include an insidious _____ *of symptoms (e.g., memory* _____, *verbal and spatial* _____*).*

The course of Alzheimer's disease tends to be gradually progressive, over the course of years.

The course of Alzheimer's disease tends to be gradually progressive, over the course of _____.

years

There may be a family history of Alzheimer's disease in those afflicted with Alzheimer's disease.

There may be a family history of Alzheimer's disease in those afflicted with _____ _____.

Alzheimer's; disease

Recent memory in those with Alzheimer's disease is worse than remote memory.

Recent memory in those with Alzheimer's disease is _____ than remote memory.

worse

Among the language deficits noted in those with Alzheimer's disease, confrontation naming tends to be problematic.

Among the language deficits noted in those with Alzheimer's disease, confrontation _____ tends to be problematic.

naming

Affective symptoms can be variable or absent in Alzheimer's disease.

Affective symptoms can be variable or _____ in Alzheimer's disease.

absent

When an individual with cognitive impairment presents with features of depression, Alzheimer's disease should be distinguished from mood disorders such as major depression.

When an individual with cognitive impairment presents with features of depression, Alzheimer's disease should be distinguished from _____ disorders such as major depression.

mood

In major depressive disorder (MDD), depressive symptoms are relatively discrete and include dysphoric mood.

In major depressive disorder (MDD), _____ symptoms are relatively discrete and include dysphoric mood.

depressive

In MDD, depression often lasts for several months if left untreated.

In MDD, depression often lasts for several _____ if left untreated.

months

In MDD, the family history is often positive for depression.

In MDD, the family _____ is often positive for depression.

history

In MDD. memory complaints tend to be patchy and inconsistent, whereas in dementia they tend to be persistent and progressive.

In _____, memory complaints tend to be patchy and inconsistent, whereas in _____ they tend to be persistent and progressive.

MDD
dementia

Patients with MDD might show increased speech latency along with depressed mood.

Patients with MDD might show increased _____ *latency along with depressed mood.*   speech

The clinical features of delirium have an abrupt onset, whereas in dementia their onset is insidious.

The clinical features of delirium have an _____   abrupt
onset, whereas in dementia their onset is _____.   insidious

Having dementia does not protect people from developing another dread condition; comorbidity is common.

Having dementia does not protect people from developing another dread condition; comorbidity is
_____.   common

When taking a history from someone with cognitive impairment, a search for disturbances of mood and psychotic symptoms should be conducted.

When taking a history from someone with cognitive impairment, a search for disturbances of mood and psychotic symptoms should be _____.   conducted

When taking the medical and surgical history of an individual with affective, behavioral, or cognitive impairment, attention should be paid to procedures and medical illnesses or conditions (e.g., head trauma), medication use, and medical symptoms.

When taking the _____ *and* _____   medical; surgical
history of an individual with affective, behavioral, or
cognitive impairment, attention should be paid to pro-
cedures and medical illnesses or conditions (e.g., head
trauma), _____ *use, and medical symptoms.*   medication

When creating a differential diagnosis for someone
with affective, behavioral, or cognitive impairment, it
is important to link neurological symptoms or signs
with different types of dementia.

When creating a differential diagnosis for someone
with affective, behavioral, or cognitive impairment,
it is important to link neurological _____ *or*   symptoms
_____ *with different types of dementia.*   signs

The presence of headache and malaise in someone
with cognitive impairment should suggest a vasculitis
or a systemic disease.

The presence of headache and malaise in someone with
cognitive impairment should suggest a _____   vasculitis
or a systemic disease.

The presence of release phenomenon (e.g., primitive
reflexes such as a grasp reflex or a snout reflex) in
someone with cognitive impairment should suggest
dementia of the Alzheimer's type or frontotemporal
lobe dementia/Pick's disease.

The presence of _____ *phenomenon (e.g., primitive* _____ *such as a grasp reflex or a snout reflex) in someone with cognitive impairment should suggest dementia of the Alzheimer's type or* _____ _____ *dementia/Pick's disease.*

The presence of long track or focal findings should raise the possibility of vascular dementia, Binswanger's encephalopathy, multiple sclerosis, HIV infection, and CNS tumors.

The presence of _____ _____ *or focal findings should raise the possibility of vascular dementia, Binswanger's encephalopathy, multiple sclerosis, HIV infection, and CNS tumors.*

The presence of EPS in someone with cognitive impairment should raise the possibility of Parkinson's disease, Huntington's disease, progressive supranuclear palsy, Wilson's disease, diffuse Lewy body disease, late-stage Alzheimer's disease, and dementia of the Alzheimer's type.

The presence of _____ *in someone with cognitive impairment should raise the possibility of Parkinson's disease, Huntington's disease, progressive supranuclear palsy, Wilson's disease, diffuse* _____ _____ *disease, late-stage Alzheimer's disease, and dementia of the Alzheimer's type.*

When incontinence and ataxia are noted in someone with cognitive impairment, a diagnosis of normal pressure hydrocephalus should be considered.

When incontinence and ataxia are noted in some-one with cognitive impairment, a diagnosis of _____ _____ hydrocephalus should be considered.

normal; pressure

Dementia is associated with a variety of degenerative conditions; for example, dementia of the Alzheimer's type, frontal lobe dementia, Pick's disease, diffuse Lewy body disease, Huntington's disease, Wilson's disease, Parkinson's disease, and progressive supranuclear palsy.

Dementia is associated with a variety of _____ conditions; for example, dementia of the Alzheimer's type, frontal lobe dementia, Pick's disease, diffuse Lewy body disease, Huntington's disease, Wilson's disease, Parkinson's disease, and progressive supranuclear palsy.

degenerative

When depression is severe, cognitive impairment can lead to the pseudodementia of depression, which improves with an upturn of the patient's mood.

When depression is severe, cognitive impairment can lead to the _____ of depression, which improves with an upturn of the patient's mood.

pseudodementia

Vascular etiologies of chronic cognitive impairment include Binswanger's encephalopathy, amyloid dementia, and diffuse ischemic injury.

Vascular etiologies of chronic cognitive impairment include Binswanger's _____, amyloid dementia, and diffuse ischemic injury.

Obstructive causes of chronic cognitive impairment include normal pressure hydrocephalus and obstructive hydrocephalus.

Obstructive causes of chronic cognitive impairment include _____ _____ hydrocephalus and obstructive hydrocephalus.

Traumatic etiologies of chronic cognitive impairment include chronic subdural hematomas, dementia pugilistica, and post-concussive syndrome.

Traumatic etiologies of chronic cognitive impairment include chronic _____ hematomas, dementia _____, and post-_____ syndrome.

Neoplastic conditions associated with chronic cognitive impairment include malignant tumors, benign tumors in the CNS (e.g., frontal lobe meningiomas), and paraneoplastic encephalitis.

_____ conditions associated with chronic cognitive impairment include malignant tumors, benign tumors in the CNS (e.g., frontal lobe meningiomas), and paraneoplastic encephalitis.

Infectious conditions that can lead to cognitive impairment include chronic meningitis (as occurs with tuberculosis), focal cerebritis, cerebral abscesses, HIV dementia, neurosyphilis, Lyme disease, and subacute sclerosing panencephalitis, Creutzfeldt-Jacob disease, and progressive multifocal leukoencephalopathy.

_____ conditions that can lead to cognitive impairment include chronic meningitis (as occurs with tuberculosis), focal cerebritis, cerebral abscesses, HIV dementia, neurosyphilis, Lyme disease, and subacute sclerosing panencephalitis, _____-Jacob disease, and progressive multifocal _____.

Infectious

Creutzfeldt-leukoencephalopathy

Demyelinating conditions such as multiple sclerosis and metachromatic leukodystrophy can also lead to chronic cognitive impairment.

_____ conditions such as multiple sclerosis and metachromatic leukodystrophy can also lead to chronic _____ impairment.

Demyelinating

cognitive

Autoimmune conditions such as systemic lupus erythematosus and polyarteritis nodosa can also lead to cognitive impairment.

Autoimmune conditions such as systemic lupus _____ and polyarteritis _____ can also lead to cognitive impairment.

erythematosus; nodosa

Substance use and abuse (e.g., alcohol, inhalants) can impair cognitive function.

Substance use and abuse (e.g., alcohol, _____) can impair cognitive function.

inhalants

A variety of medications (including anticholinergic agents and beta-blockers) can impair cognition.

A variety of medications (including _____ agents and _____-blockers) can impair cognition.

anticholinergic
beta-

A bevy of toxins, such as arsenic, bromide, carbon monoxide, mercury, and organophosphates, can impair cognitive function.

A bevy of toxins, such as arsenic, bromide, carbon _____, mercury, and organophosphates, can impair _____ function.

monoxide
cognitive

The mental status examination, which is a subset of the comprehensive physical examination, is essential in the search for disturbances in affect, behavior, and cognition.

The _____ _____ examination, which is a subset of the comprehensive physical examination, is essential in the search for disturbances in affect, behavior, and cognition.

mental; status

Adjuncts to the mental status examination include bedside cognitive tests such as the "draw-a-clock" test, a task involving copying simple designs or patterns (e.g., 0+0++0+++0++++), and asking the patient to perform simple tasks to test praxis (e.g., make the motion you would use to comb your hair or brush your teeth).

Adjuncts to the mental status examination include bedside _____ tests such as the "draw-a-_____" test, a task involving copying simple designs or _____ (e.g., 0+0++0+++0++++), and asking the patient to perform simple tasks to test _____ (e.g., make the motion you would use to comb your hair or brush your teeth).

cognitive
clock
patterns

praxis

Impairments in performance when drawing the numbers of a clock and setting the hands of the clock to "ten to two" include poor planning of spacing between the numbers, perseveration (e.g., repeating some numbers, or not having the hour hand and minute hand meet at the center of the clock face, and instead meeting above the clock's center [leading to a suggestion that the individual is stimulus-bound, and "pulled" to the numbers 10 and 2]).

Impairments in performance when drawing the numbers of a clock and setting the hands of the clock to "ten to two" include _____ _____ of spacing between the numbers, _____ (e.g., repeating some numbers, or not having the hour hand and minute hand meet at the center of the clock face, and instead meeting above the clock's center [leading to a suggestion that the individual is _____- _____, and "pulled" to the numbers 10 and 2]).

poor; planning
perseveration

stimulus-
bound

Formal neuropsychiatric testing batteries can provide detailed assessments of cognitive function and impairment.

Formal _____ _____ batteries can provide detailed assessments of cognitive function and impairment.

neuropsychiatric; testing

If an electroencephalogram (EEG) is obtained, it is usually abnormal in a delirious patient.

If an electroencephalogram (EEG) is obtained, it is usually _____ in a delirious patient.

abnormal

If an EEG is obtained in a delirious patient, it usually demonstrates diffuse, generalized slowing.

If an EEG is obtained in a delirious patient, it usually demonstrates diffuse, _____ _____.

Generalized slowing on an EEG of a delirious patient is a non-specific finding.

Generalized _____ on an EEG of a delirious patient is a non-_____ finding.

Summary

Being delirious can negatively affect health care outcomes, for example, more frequent falls, increased length of stay, institutionalization after discharge, decline in functional status, and cognitive decline.

Being delirious can negatively affect health care outcomes, for example, more frequent _____, increased length of _____, institutionalization after _____, _____ in functional status, and _____ decline.

Delirium is a highly prevalent condition; it occurs in roughly 30% of general hospital inpatients, 60% of elderly general hospital inpatients, and up to 80% of ICU patients.

Delirium is a highly prevalent condition; it occurs in roughly 30% of general hospital inpatients, 60% of elderly general hospital inpatients, and up to _____% of ICU patients.

Early recognition of the risk factors for the diagnosis of delirium is essential for the prevention of delirium and for timely treatment of delirium, when it develops.

Early recognition of the risk factors for the diagnosis of _____ is essential for the _____ of delirium and for timely _____ of delirium, when it develops.

delirium; prevention
treatment

Despite the importance of early diagnosis and risk stratification, delirium is typically under-diagnosed and under-reported.

Despite the importance of early _____ and risk _____, delirium is typically under-_____ and under-_____.

diagnosis
stratification
diagnosed; reported

Delirium is a preventable and treatable source of substantial morbidity.

Delirium is a _____ and treatable source of substantial _____.

preventable
morbidity

Diagnosis of delirium is a precondition of its treatment.

_____ of delirium is a precondition of its treatment.

Diagnosis

Accurate identification of risk factors for delirium is an important first step to targeting prevention efforts.

Accurate identification of risk _____ for delirium is an important first step to targeting prevention efforts.

factors

Laboratory studies that contribute to our understanding of the etiology of cognitive deficits include routine blood tests.

Laboratory studies that contribute to our understanding of the etiology of cognitive deficits include routine _____ tests.

blood

Blood tests obtained during the assessment of impaired cognition include a complete blood count, levels of vitamin B_{12} and folate, sedimentation rate, and levels of glucose, calcium, phosphorus, magnesium, as well as electrolytes.

Blood tests obtained during the assessment of impaired cognition include a complete _____ count, levels of vitamin B_{12} and folate, sedimentation _____, and levels of glucose, calcium, phosphorus, magnesium, as well as electrolytes.

blood

rate

Blood tests obtained during the assessment of cognitive impairment also include tests of liver, thyroid, and kidney function, as well as a syphilis serology (or RPR).

Blood tests obtained during the assessment of cognitive impairment also include tests of liver, _____, and kidney function, as well as a _____ serology (or RPR).

thyroid
syphilis

Urine tests and other laboratory studies include an electrocardiogram, a CT or MRI scan, a chest X-ray, and EEG, noninvasive carotid studies, HIV testing, rheumatoid factor and antinuclear antibodies (ANA), CSF analysis, drug levels, and heavy metal screening.

Urine tests and other laboratory studies include an elec-
trocardiogram, a CT or MRI scan, a chest X-ray, and
EEG, noninvasive carotid studies, HIV testing, rheu-
matoid factor and antinuclear _____ (ANA),   antibodies
CSF analysis, drug levels, and heavy _____   metal
screening.

Findings of the mental status examination, a comprehensive history and physical examination, and laboratory assessment should be considered in the context
of a timeline for symptom development and illness
course.

Findings of the mental status examination, a compre-
hensive history and physical examination, and labora-
tory assessment should be considered in the context of
a _____ for symptom development and illness   timeline
course.

Although clinicians try to find a unifying hypothesis
to explain all signs and symptoms (i.e., using "Occam's
razor"), they must also realize that a patient can have
as many conditions as they please (i.e., "Hickam's
dictum").

Although clinicians try to find a unifying hypoth-
esis to explain all signs and symptoms (i.e., using
"_____"), they must also realize that a patient   Occam's razor
can have as many conditions as they please (i.e.,
"_____").   Hickam's dictum

Post-Reading Quiz

Post-Reading Quiz: Answer Sheet

1. _____
2. _____
3. _____
4. _____
5. _____
6. _____
7. _____
8. _____
9. _____
10. _____
11. _____
12. _____
13. _____
14. _____
15. _____
16. _____
17. _____
18. _____
19. _____
20. _____

21. _____

22. _____

23. _____

24. _____

25. _____

26. _____

27. _____

28. _____

29. _____

30. _____

31. _____

32. _____

33. _____

34. _____

35. _____

36. _____

37. _____

38. _____

39. _____

40. _____

41. _____

42. _____

43. _____

44. _____

45. _____

46. _____

47. _____

48. _____

49. _____

50. _____

Post-Reading Quiz: Questions

1. Which of the following is the best term to describe a clinician's bedside assessment of affect, behavior, and cognition?
   A. Disability assessment
   B. Mental status examination
   C. Neuropsychiatric testing
   D. Physical examination

2. Which of the following is assessed when a clinician observes how a patient appears?
   A. Affect
   B. Cognition
   C. Judgment
   D. Mood

3. Which of the following is assessed when a clinician asks a patient how they are feeling?
   A. Affect
   B. Cognition
   C. Judgment
   D. Mood

4. Acute brain failure is most closely related to which of the following terms?
   A. Binswanger's encephalopathy
   B. Delirium
   C. Dementia
   D. Seizures

5. Chronic brain failure is most closely related to which of the following terms?
   A. Delirium
   B. Dementia
   C. Hypoglycemia
   D. Seizures

6. Which of the following features is characteristic of delirium?
   A. Abulia
   B. Agnosia
   C. Aphasia
   D. Disorientation

7. Which of the following features is characteristic of delirium?
   A. Impaired attention and concentration
   B. Non-fluent aphasia
   C. Nystagmus
   D. Word-finding difficulty

8. Which of the following features is characteristic of delirium?
   A. Negativism
   B. Perceptual disturbances
   C. Staring spells
   D. Waxy flexibility

9. Paranoid ideas are an example of which of the following?
   A. Thought blocking
   B. Thought broadcasting
   C. Thought content
   D. Thought process

10. Which of the following terms best describes excessive, non-purposeful motor activity?
    A. Agitation
    B. Catatonia
    C. Delirium
    D. Psychosis

11. Which of the following terms is used to describe the task of asking a patient to subtract the number seven sequentially from 100?
    A. Concrete thinking
    B. Executive function
    C. Planning
    D. Serial sevens

12. Which of the following is the domain tested by asking a patient to spell the word "WORLD" backward?
    A. Abulia
    B. Attention and concentration
    C. Broca's aphasia
    D. Wernicke's aphasia

13. Which of the following is a brief test of cognition?
    A. HAM-D
    B. MMPI
    C. MMSE
    D. PHQ-9

14. Which of the following is a brief test of cognition?

   A. MoCA

   B. PAI

   C. WAIS

   D. WCST

15. Which of the following is a brief test of cognition?

   A. BPRS

   B. CAM-ICU

   C. CGI

   D. MINI

16. On average, how many minutes does it take to administer the MMSE?

   A. Less than two

   B. 5 to 10

   C. 15 to 20

   D. 45 to 60

17. Which of the following is a normal score on the MoCA?

   A. Less than 10

   B. 10 to 15

   C. 20 to 25

   D. More than 26

18. Which of the following can be assessed by poor placement of numbers when a patient is asked to draw a clock?

   A. Aprosodia

   B. Broca's aphasia

   C. Executive dysfunction

   D. Wernicke's syndrome

19. Which of the following terms describes seeing something that isn't there?
    A. A delusion
    B. A hallucination
    C. An illusion
    D. A paranoid belief

20. Which of the following terms would best describe the experience of a patient with a Foley catheter, when he tells you that he sees a snake sitting on his leg?
    A. A delusion
    B. A hallucination
    C. An illusion
    D. A paranoid belief

21. Which of the following is the most important determinant of the treatment of the agitated and delirious patient?
    A. Age of the patient
    B. Cost of the treatment
    C. Etiology of the delirium
    D. Prognosis of the patient

22. Which of the following is the *least* helpful term in establishing an etiology of delirium?
    A. Hypoglycemia
    B. Hypponatremia
    C. Hypoxemia
    D. ICU psychosis

23. Which of the following terms is most synonymous with word "delirious"?

    A. Agitated

    B. Encephalopathic

    C. Paranoid

    D. Psychotic

24. Which of the following is a characteristic feature of delirium?

    A. Fever

    B. Fluctuations

    C. Paranoia

    D. Persistence

25. Which of the following best describes a fixed, false belief?

    A. A delusion

    B. An illusion

    C. A hallucination

    D. Paranoia

26. Which of the following is most closely associated with the development of mania?

    A. Beta blockers

    B. Calcium channel-blockers

    C. Corticosteroids

    D. NSAIDs

27. Which of the following mnemonics can be used to recall the life-threatening causes of delirium?

    A. DIGFAST

    B. DTRHIGH

    C. SIGECAPS

    D. WWHHHHIIMMPS

28. The triad of ataxia, confusion, and ophthalmoplegia is highly suggestive of which of the following conditions?

    A. Catatonia

    B. Delirium

    C. Serotonin syndrome

    D. Wernicke's encephalopathy

29. Which of the following would be most likely if a patient demonstrates confusion, tachycardia, mydriasis, reduced bowel sounds, dry skin, and flushing?

    A. Adrenergic excess

    B. Anticholinergic delirium

    C. Hypoglycemia

    D. Narcotic withdrawal

30. Which of the following can reverse many of the manifestations of an amitriptyline overdose?

    A. Atropine

    B. Flumazenil

    C. Naloxone

    D. Physostigmine

31. Deficiency of which of the following substances would be likely to lead to Wernicke's encephalopathy?

    A. Folic acid

    B. Niacin

    C. Thiamine

    D. Vitamin B_{12}

32. Benzodiazepines with which of the following half-lives are most likely to lead to a withdrawal syndrome after sudden discontinuation or a dramatic decrease in the dose?

A. Less than three hours

B. 5 to 10 hours

C. 10 to 20 hours

D. More than 40 hours

33. Which of the following routes of administration of haloperidol is likely to lead to the lowest risk of acute extrapyramidal symptoms?

A. Intramuscular

B. Intravenous

C. Oral

D. Transdermal patch

34. Dementia is a syndrome characterized by a clinically significant decline in memory as well as by at least one of the following domains?

A. Ambulation

B. Appetite

C. Higher cortical function

D. Mood

35. Dementia usually develops over which of the following time periods?

A. Minutes to hours

B. Days to weeks

C. Weeks to months

D. Months to years

36. Dementia is manifest by which of the following?
    A. A tripling of the prevalence every five years beyond the age of 60
    B. An acquired decline in memory
    C. An irreversible loss of memory
    D. Weight gain

37. The prevalence of dementia in individuals above the age of 60 is which of the following?
    A. 1%
    B. 5%
    C. 15%
    D. 50%

38. The prevalence of dementia at age 60 is which of the following?
    A. 1%
    B. 5%
    C. 15%
    D. 50%

39. The prevalence of dementia among those aged 85 is which of the following?
    A. 5%
    B. 15%
    C. 50%
    D. 75%

40. In which of the following conditions is there an autosomal dominant pattern of inheritance of dementia?
    A. Diffuse Lewy body disease
    B. Huntington's disease
    C. Multiple sclerosis
    D. Parkinson's disease

41. Which of the following types of dementia is associated with a step-wise decline in function?
    A. Alzheimer's disease
    B. Diffuse Lewy body disease
    C. Parkinson's disease
    D. Vascular dementia

42. Which of the following is identified as an activity of daily living?
    A. Toileting
    B. Managing money
    C. Shopping
    D. Using the telephone

43. Which of the following is identified as an instrumental activity of daily living?
    A. Bathing
    B. Dressing
    C. Feeding
    D. Preparing meals

44. Which of the following statements about Alzheimer's disease is *true*?
    A. Afflicted patients are not allowed to sign contracts
    B. Remote memory is worse than recent memory
    C. Symptom onset is abrupt
    D. The course is gradually progressive

45. The presence of headache and malaise in someone with cognitive impairment should suggest which of the following conditions?
    A. A degenerative disease
    B. Obstructive hydrocephalus
    C. Pseudodementia
    D. Vasculitis

46. The presence of ataxia, incontinence, and confusion should suggest which of the following conditions?
    A. AIDS
    B. Normal pressure hydrocephalus
    C. Parkinson's disease
    D. Syphilis

47. The presence of extrapyramidal symptoms should suggest which of the following conditions?
    A. Alzheimer's disease
    B. Diffuse Lewy body disease
    C. Normal pressure hydrocephalus
    D. Vitamin B$_{12}$ deficiency

48. Which of the following is an autoimmune disorder associated with cognitive impairment?
    A. Creutzfeldt-Jacob disease
    B. Lyme disease
    C. Neurosyphilis
    D. Systemic lupus erythematosus

49. Which of the following is a brief bedside cognitive screening test?

    A. "Draw-a-clock" test

    B. HAM-D

    C. SCID

    D. YBOCS

50. Which of the following is the phrase associated with the concept that a patient can have multiple simultaneous conditions?

    A. Bernoulli's theorem

    B. Hickam's dictum

    C. Markovnikov's rule

    D. Occam's razor

Post-Reading Quiz: Answer Key

Note: This answer key should be viewed after taking the pre-test, reading the text, and taking the post-reading quiz.

1. _____B_____

2. _____A_____

3. _____D_____

4. _____B_____

5. _____B_____

6. _____D_____

7. _____A_____

8. _____B_____

9. _____C_____

10. _____A_____

11. _____D_____

12. _____B_____

13. _____C_____

14. _____A_____

15. _____B_____

16. _____B_____

17. _____D_____

18. _____C_____

19. _____B_____

20. _____C_____

Answers continued on next page.

21. _____C_____

22. _____D_____

23. _____B_____

24. _____B_____

25. _____A_____

26. _____C_____

27. _____D_____

28. _____D_____

29. _____B_____

30. _____D_____

31. _____C_____

32. _____C_____

33. _____B_____

34. _____C_____

35. _____D_____

36. _____B_____

37. _____C_____

38. _____A_____

39. _____C_____

40. _____B_____

41. _____D_____

42. _____A_____

43. _____D_____

44. _____D_____

45. _____D_____

46. _____B_____

47. _____B_____

48. _____D_____

49. _____A_____

50. _____B_____

PRE-TEST SCORE:
_____ (Number of correct answers)
_____ (Percent of correct answers)

POST-READING SCORE:
_____ (Number of correct answers)
_____ (Percent of correct answers)

Post-Reading Quiz: Answers

1. Which of the following is the best term to describe a clinician's bedside assessment of affect, behavior, and cognition?
   A. Disability assessment
   B. **Mental status examination**
   C. Neuropsychiatric testing
   D. Physical examination

2. Which of the following is assessed when a clinician observes how a patient appears?
   A. **Affect**
   B. Cognition
   C. Judgment
   D. Mood

3. Which of the following is assessed when a clinician asks a patient how they are feeling?
   A. Affect
   B. Cognition
   C. Judgment
   D. **Mood**

4. Acute brain failure is most closely related to which of the following terms?
   A. Binswanger's encephalopathy
   B. **Delirium**
   C. Dementia
   D. Seizures

5. Chronic brain failure is most closely related to which of the following terms?

    A. Delirium
    B. **Dementia**
    C. Hypoglycemia
    D. Seizures

6. Which of the following features is characteristic of delirium?

    A. Abulia
    B. Agnosia
    C. Aphasia
    D. **Disorientation**

7. Which of the following features is characteristic of delirium?

    A. **Impaired attention and concentration**
    B. Non-fluent aphasia
    C. Nystagmus
    D. Word-finding difficulty

8. Which of the following features is characteristic of delirium?

    A. Negativism
    B. **Perceptual disturbances**
    C. Staring spells
    D. Waxy flexibility

9. Paranoid ideas are an example of which of the following?

    A. Thought blocking
    B. Thought broadcasting
    C. **Thought content**
    D. Thought process

10. Which of the following terms best describes excessive, non-purposeful motor activity?

    A. **Agitation**

    B. Catatonia

    C. Delirium

    D. Psychosis

11. Which of the following terms is used to describe the task of asking a patient to subtract the number seven sequentially from 100?

    A. Concrete thinking

    B. Executive function

    C. Planning

    D. **Serial sevens**

12. Which of the following is the domain tested by asking a patient to spell the word "WORLD" backward?

    A. Abulia

    B. **Attention and concentration**

    C. Broca's aphasia

    D. Wernicke's aphasia

13. Which of the following is a brief test of cognition?

    A. HAM-D

    B. MMPI

    C. **MMSE**

    D. PHQ-9

14. Which of the following is a brief test of cognition?
    A. **MoCA**
    B. PAI
    C. WAIS
    D. WCST

15. Which of the following is a brief test of cognition?
    A. BPRS
    B. **CAM-ICU**
    C. CGI
    D. MINI

16. On average, how many minutes does it take to administer the MMSE?
    A. Less than two
    B. **5 to 10**
    C. 15 to 20
    D. 45 to 60

17. Which of the following is a normal score on the MoCA?
    A. Less than 10
    B. 10 to 15
    C. 20 to 25
    D. **More than 26**

18. Which of the following can be assessed by poor placement of numbers when a patient is asked to draw a clock?
    A. Aprosodia
    B. Broca's aphasia
    C. **Executive dysfunction**
    D. Wernicke's syndrome

19. Which of the following terms describes seeing something that isn't there?

    A. A delusion

    B. **A hallucination**

    C. An illusion

    D. A paranoid belief

20. Which of the following terms would best describe the experience of a patient with a Foley catheter, when he tells you that he sees a snake sitting on his leg?

    A. A delusion

    B. A hallucination

    C. **An illusion**

    D. A paranoid belief

21. Which of the following is the most important determinant of the treatment of the agitated and delirious patient?

    A. Age of the patient

    B. Cost of the treatment

    C. **Etiology of the delirium**

    D. Prognosis of the patient

22. Which of the following is the least helpful term in establishing an etiology of delirium?

    A. Hypoglycemia

    B. Hypponatremia

    C. Hypoxemia

    D. **ICU psychosis**

23. Which of the following terms is most synonymous with word "delirious"?
    A. Agitated
    B. **Encephalopathic**
    C. Paranoid
    D. Psychotic

24. Which of the following is a characteristic feature of delirium?
    A. Fever
    B. **Fluctuations**
    C. Paranoia
    D. Persistence

25. Which of the following best describes a fixed, false belief?
    A. **A delusion**
    B. An illusion
    C. A hallucination
    D. Paranoia

26. Which of the following is most closely associated with the development of mania?
    A. Beta blockers
    B. Calcium channel-blockers
    C. **Corticosteroids**
    D. NSAIDs

27. Which of the following mnemonics can be used to recall the life-threatening causes of delirium?
    A. DIGFAST
    B. DTRHIGH
    C. SIGECAPS
    D. **WWHHHHIIMMPS**

28. The triad of ataxia, confusion, and ophthalmoplegia is highly suggestive of which of the following conditions?

    A. Catatonia

    B. Delirium

    C. Serotonin syndrome

    D. **Wernicke's encephalopathy**

29. Which of the following would be most likely if a patient demonstrates confusion, tachycardia, mydriasis, reduced bowel sounds, dry skin, and flushing?

    A. Adrenergic excess

    B. **Anticholinergic delirium**

    C. Hypoglycemia

    D. Narcotic withdrawal

30. Which of the following can reverse many of the manifestations of an amitriptyline overdose?

    A. Atropine

    B. Flumazenil

    C. Naloxone

    D. **Physostigmine**

31. Deficiency of which of the following substances would be likely to lead to Wernicke's encephalopathy?

    A. Folic acid

    B. Niacin

    C. **Thiamine**

    D. Vitamin B_{12}

32. Benzodiazepines with which of the following half-lives are most likely to lead to a withdrawal syndrome after sudden discontinuation or a dramatic decrease in the dose?
   A. Less than three hours
   B. 5 to 10 hours
   C. **10 to 20 hours**
   D. More than 40 hours

33. Which of the following routes of administration of haloperidol is likely to lead to the lowest risk of acute extrapyramidal symptoms?
   A. Intramuscular
   B. **Intravenous**
   C. Oral
   D. Transdermal patch

34. Dementia is a syndrome characterized by a clinically significant decline in memory as well as by at least one of the following domains?
   A. Ambulation
   B. Appetite
   C. **Higher cortical function**
   D. Mood

35. Dementia usually develops over which of the following time periods?
   A. Minutes to hours
   B. Days to weeks
   C. Weeks to months
   D. **Months to years**

36. Dementia is manifest by which of the following?

    A. A tripling of the prevalence every five years beyond the age of 60

    B. **An acquired decline in memory**

    C. An irreversible loss of memory

    D. Weight gain

37. The prevalence of dementia in individuals above the age of 60 is which of the following?

    A. 1%

    B. 5%

    C. **15%**

    D. 50%

38. The prevalence of dementia at age 60 is which of the following?

    A. **1%**

    B. 5%

    C. 15%

    D. 50%

39. The prevalence of dementia among those aged 85 is which of the following?

    A. 5%

    B. 15%

    C. **50%**

    D. 75%

40. In which of the following conditions is there an autosomal dominant pattern of inheritance of dementia?

   A. Diffuse Lewy body disease

   B. **Huntington's disease**

   C. Multiple sclerosis

   D. Parkinson's disease

41. Which of the following types of dementia is associated with a step-wise decline in function?

   A. Alzheimer's disease

   B. Diffuse Lewy body disease

   C. Parkinson's disease

   D. **Vascular dementia**

42. Which of the following is identified as an activity of daily living?

   A. **Toileting**

   B. Managing money

   C. Shopping

   D. Using the telephone

43. Which of the following is identified as an instrumental activity of daily living?

   A. Bathing

   B. Dressing

   C. Feeding

   D. **Preparing meals**

44. Which of the following statements about Alzheimer's disease is *true*?

   A. Afflicted patients are not allowed to sign contracts

   B. Remote memory is worse than recent memory

   C. Symptom onset is abrupt

   D. **The course is gradually progressive**

45. The presence of headache and malaise in someone with cognitive impairment should suggest which of the following conditions?

   A. A degenerative disease

   B. Obstructive hydrocephalus

   C. Pseudodementia

   D. **Vasculitis**

46. The presence of ataxia, incontinence, and confusion should suggest which of the following conditions?

   A. AIDS

   B. **Normal pressure hydrocephalus**

   C. Parkinson's disease

   D. Syphilis

47. The presence of extrapyramidal symptoms should suggest which of the following conditions?

   A. Alzheimer's disease

   B. **Diffuse Lewy body disease**

   C. Normal pressure hydrocephalus

   D. Vitamin B_{12} deficiency

48. Which of the following is an autoimmune disorder associated with cognitive impairment?

   A. Creutzfeldt-Jacob disease

   B. Lyme disease

   C. Neurosyphilis

   D. **Systemic lupus erythematosus**

49. Which of the following is a brief bedside cognitive screening test?

    A. **"Draw-a-clock" test**

    B. HAM-D

    C. SCID

    D. YBOCS

50. Which of the following is the phrase associated with the concept that a patient can have multiple simultaneous conditions?

    A. Bernoulli's theorem

    B. **Hickam's dictum**

    C. Markovnikov's rule

    D. Occam's razor

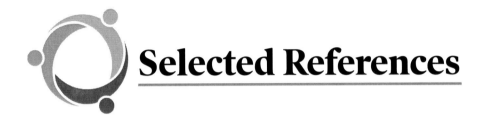

Selected References

1. Cremens MC: Geriatric psychiatry. In: Stern TA, Fava M, Wilens TE, et al, eds.: *Massachusetts General Hospital Comprehensive Clinical Psychiatry*. 2nd ed.: Philadelphia, PA: Elsevier; 2016: 763–769.

2. Falk W: The patient with memory problems or dementia. In: Stern TA, Herman JB, Slavin PL, eds.: *The MGH Guide to Psychiatry in Primary Care*. 6th ed.: New York: McGraw-Hill; 2004: 197–212.

3. Falk WE, Wiechers IR: Demented patients. In: Stern TA, Fricchione GL, Cassem NH, et al, eds.: *Massachusetts General Hospital Handbook of General Hospital Psychiatry*. 6th ed.: Philadelphia, PA: Elsevier; 2010: 105–118.

4. Gatchel JR, Wright CI, Falk WE, et al: Dementia. In: Stern TA, Fava M, Wilens TE, et al, eds.: *Massachusetts General Hospital Comprehensive Clinical Psychiatry*. 2nd ed.: Philadelphia, PA: Elsevier; 2016: 184–197.

5. Heckers S, Tesar GE, Querques J, et al: Diagnosis and treatment of agitation and delirium in the intensive care unit patient. In: Irwin RS, Rippe JM, eds.: *Intensive Care Medicine*. 5th ed.: Philadelphia, PA: Lippincott-Williams & Wilkins; 2003, 2153–2162.

6. Larsen KA, Kelly SE, Stern TA, et al: Administration of olanzapine to prevent postoperative delirium in elderly joint replacement patients: a randomized controlled study. *Psychosomatics*. 2010; 51: 409–418.

7. Stern TA, Celano CM, Gross AF, et al: The assessment and management of agitation and delirium in the general hospital. *Prim Care Companion J Clin Psychiatry.* 2012; 12(1): e1–e11.

8. Stern TA, Herman JB, Slavin PL, eds.: *The MGH Guide to Primary Care Psychiatry.* 2nd ed.: New York: McGraw-Hill; 2004.

9. Stern TA, Freudenreich O, Smith FA, et al, eds.: *Massachusetts General Hospital Handbook of General Hospital Psychiatry.* 7th ed.: Philadelphia, PA: Saunders/Elsevier; 2018.

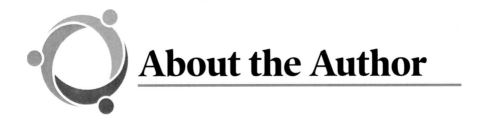

About the Author

Theodore A. Stern, MD is the Ned H. Cassem Professor of Psychiatry in the field of Psychosomatic Medicine/Consultation, Harvard Medical School and Chief Emeritus of the Avery D. Weisman Psychiatry Consultation Service, the Director of the Thomas P. Hackett Center for Scholarship in Psychosomatic Medicine, and the Director of the Office for Clinical Careers at the Massachusetts General Hospital in Boston, Massachusetts. Dr. Stern has written more than 450 scientific articles and book chapters and edited more than 25 books. These include: *Massachusetts General Hospital Handbook of General Hospital Psychiatry* (4/e–7/e); *Massachusetts General Hospital Comprehensive Clinical Psychiatry* (1/e, 2/e); *Massachusetts General Hospital Guide to Primary Care Psychiatry* (1/e, 2/e); *Massachusetts General Hospital Psychiatry Update & Board Preparations* (1/e–4/e); *Facing Cancer; Facing Heart Disease; Facing Diabetes; Facing Immunotherapy; Facing Scleroderma; Facing Lupus; Facing Osteoporosis; Facing Rheumatoid Arthritis; Facing Cystic Fibrosis; Facing Psoriasis;* and *Facing Overweight and Obesity; Learning About the Assessment and Management of Suicide Risk; Learning About Factitious Illness and Malingering; Learning About Catatonia, Neuroleptic Malignant Syndrome, and Serotonin Syndrome; Learning About Informed Consent, Capacity Assessments, Treatment Refusal, Civil Commitment, and Boundary Violations;* and *Learning About Sleep and Sleep Disorders.* He is also the editor-in-chief of *Psychosomatics.*